D0072531

# ANXIETY IN CHILDREN

# Anxiety in Children

**Edited by Ved P Varma**

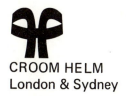

CROOM HELM
London & Sydney

METHUEN
New York

© 1984 Ved P. Varma
Croom Helm Ltd, Provident House, Burrell Row,
Beckenham, Kent BR3 1AT
Croom Helm Australia Pty Ltd, First Floor,
139 King Street, Sydney, NSW 2001, Australia

British Library Cataloguing in Publication Data

    Anxiety in children.
    1. Anxiety in children,
    I. Varma, Ved P.
    618.92′85223        RJ506.A58
    ISBN 0-7099-2607-3

Published in the United States of America by
Methuen, Inc., 733 Third Avenue, New York,
N.Y. 10017

Library of Congress Cataloging in Publication Data

Main entry under title:
    Anxiety in children.

    Bibliography: P.
    Includes index.
    1. Anxiety in children.   I. Varma, Ved P.
BF723.A5A59   1984     618.92′85223   84-1173
ISBN 0-416-01031-8

Printed and bound in Great Britain

# CONTENTS

*To my daughter, who never made me more anxious
than she had to.*

Ved Varma

# CONTRIBUTORS

James W. Anderson, PhD: Tutor, London Centre for Psycho-therapy, and Psychotherapist, St Bernard's Hospital, 8 Lowther Road, London SW13 9NJ.

Philip Barker, MB, BS, FRCP(Ed), FRCPsych, FRCP(C): Professor of Psychiatry and Paediatrics, University of Calgary, Alberta Children's Hospital, 1820 Richmond Road SW, Calgary, Alberta, Canada T2T 5C7.

Lindy Burton, PhD: Consultant Psychologist, The Coachhouse, 3 Kathleen Avenue, Helen's Bay, Co. Down, Northern Ireland. Also teaches at Queen's University, Belfast, Royal Victoria Hospital, Belfast, and at Action Cancer, Belfast.

Susanna Isaacs Elmhirst, MD, MRCP, FRCP, FRCPsych: Consultant Child Psychiatrist, Child Guidance Training Centre, 120 Belsize Lane, London NW3 5BA, and Physician-in-Charge, Children's Department, Institute of Psychoanalysis, London.

Martin Herbert, PhD: Professor of Psychology, University of Leicester, University Road, Leicester LE1 7RH.

David Jones, PhD: Lecturer, Department of Psychology, Birkbeck College, University of London, Malet Street, London WC1E 7HX.

Vaman G. Lokare, BA, MA, MPhil, PhD, ABPSs: Top Grade Clinical Psychologist, West Park Hospital, Horton Lane, Epsom, Surrey KT19 8PB.

Rev. Eamonn F. O'Doherty, PhD: Catholic Priest, and Professor of Logic and Psychology, University College, Belfield, Dublin 4, Ireland.

Elsie L. Osborne, BSc: Principal Educational Psychologist, The Tavistock Clinic, 120 Belsize Lane, London NW3 5BA.

Ved P. Varma, PhD: Former Educational Psychologist, London Borough of Brent. His other books include *Stress in Children, Psychotherapy Today, Advances in Educational Psychology, 1* (co-editor W. D. Wall), *Advances in Educational Psychology, 2* (co-editor M. L. K. Pringle) and *Piaget, Psychology and Education* (co-editor Phillip Williams).

Timothy Telford Yates, BSc, MDCM, DipPsychol, FRCP(C), FAOA: Associate Professor, Departments of Psychiatry and

*Contributors*

Paediatrics, Faculty of Medicine, University of Calgary, and Head, Mental Health Program, Psychiatrist-in-Chief, Alberta Children's Hospital, 1820 Richmond Road SW, Calgary, Alberta, Canada T2T 5C7.

# INTRODUCTION

All of us have experienced anxiety at one time or another, in our personal relationships, in our work, concerning our health, or in all of these and perhaps other areas as well. It is not surprising therefore, says Sargant,[1] that in a recent three-year period in Great Britain, for instance, a staggering total of 43 million prescriptions were dispensed for psychotropic drugs to combat states of anxiety and tension in one form or another. Yet this total does not even include all the additional tranquillisers, sedatives and antidepressants used in the hundreds of general and mental hospitals in Great Britain, and also in the private practice sector of medicine and psychiatry. According to Ingleby,[2] in the USA doctors write 200 million prescriptions for psychoactive drugs in the course of a single year.

Thus anxiety is a matter of great current concern. We are living in an age of anxiety. But it is not only adults who experience the problem. Indeed, it can be argued that anxiety is most evident during periods of rapid change. And since childhood is the period during which we develop most rapidly, then a strong case can be made for anxiety being especially prevalent in children.

This book gives a broad discussion by well-known experts of the issues of anxiety in children, focusing particularly on what those involved in mental health and educational and clinical psychology, can do to help. I hope the content is interesting. I hope that every reader will take the book for what it is worth and compare it with the fruits of his or her own wisdom and experience. Finally, may those who read this book come to realise that the world belongs to those who work for those less fortunate than themselves.

The editor would like to thank the reader for taking the trouble to read this book. As regards my publishing colleagues David Croom and Tim Hardwick, and the contributors to this book, it is impossible to express my deep gratitude in words — it is implied in working in partnership with them in this context.

Ved Varma

*Introduction*

## References

1. Sargant, William, 'Physical Treatment of Anxiety' in M. H. Lader (ed.), *Studies in Anxiety* (World Psychiatric Association 1969).
2. Ingleby, David (ed.), *Critical Psychiatry* (Penguin, Harmondsworth, 1981).

# 1 A PSYCHOANALYTIC APPROACH TO ANXIETY IN CHILDHOOD

Susanna Isaacs Elmhirst

Most adults experience some conscious anxiety in their day-to-day lives, usually they can call to mind some of their own childhood fears. Yet there are a few grown-ups who are not at all aware of suffering fear or nervousness in situations when such a response might very well be expected. This unawareness would generally be recognised as abnormal. An extreme example is a woman who was quite unperturbed by being afflicted with paralysis of one limb. It is possible that some people would regard such lack of response as courage and congratulate the victim. But most of us would support a friend in such a plight in seeking help, even perhaps from a psychoanalyst, if no organic cause could be found for the loss of limb power. If recovery of movement was accompanied by the regaining of emotional mobility, as with one of Freud's[1] early patients, both changes would ordinarily be welcomed as signs of improved mental health. Yet there are many adults who seriously believe that anxiety in children is all pathological and preventable. It follows that people who hold this view are pleased, not concerned, when a child shows no fear in frightening circumstances. The motives of these adults are, of course, complex. An important source of their inability to see anxiety when it is obviously manifested by children is their praiseworthy wish to make young people happy. Such an aim is not uncommonly linked with an adult's wish to feel him or herself to be a good and kind person.

Children manifest their anxiety in ways which are often the same as in adults and which would ordinarily be recognised in, and by, adults. They say they suffer and tell us, in words, why. They want to run away or escape somehow. They will tell us so or try to achieve their aim, freedom from fear, sometimes even to the point of destroying themselves. They quake or tremble, weep, wet themselves. They may vomit or go very pale. People who cannot see that children behaving in one or more of these ways are suffering from fear are going to be in greater difficulty when it comes to the more subtly revealed manifestations of a child's unconscious anxiety.

1

But of course adults who are so blind to children's fears will not see that they, themselves, are in difficulties. They may even say or imply proudly, like the headmistress of a school attended by one of my patients, '*we* don't have any unhappy children in this school'.

When he embarked on the 'talking cure' Freud found that if his patients could express themselves freely in words he could perceive themes and motives of which the sufferers were unaware. In the setting that he provided Freud perceived that these feelings were spontaneously concentrated upon him. He also found that when he described, in words to the patient, what he could see of the emotional patterns and their origins, the patient could sometimes comprehend as well. A further finding was that the self-knowledge obtained by Freud's 'analysis' of the sufferer's communications could, on occasion, give relief to the patient. But relief of anxiety and of mental pain led to the release of more emotional experiences of which the patient had been previously unaware. These too were then available for study. As these more deeply hidden feelings emerged they also were liable to cause the patient conscious, and at times intense, mental suffering. Freud then came to realise that the original symptoms were often an attempt by the patient to protect himself from unbearable emotional experiences. But that protection was gained at such a cost that all search for relief had previously proved unsuccessful.

During the early part of his long working-life as a psychoanalyst Freud was impressed by the intensity and diversity of childhood sexual feelings that were re-captured in his adult consulting-room, with himself as their object. He described these patients as 'transferring' their feelings, from the original people who had stimulated them, on to himself as analyst. Many adult patients felt and thought that they had in childhood been sexually seduced by adults. For a time Freud also believed that they all had actually had such physical experiences. Then he began to see that the vivid sense of such an experience could also arise in the imagination; in other words in the 'fantasy' life of the patients. From then on Freud was even more fascinated and absorbed by the workings of what he called the unconscious mind. Not only was it a store-house for memories of real, external events and justified rational feelings, but also a treasure trove of fantasies, some of which had obviously been active since early childhood, which were different from the conscious day-dreams of which we all know. So Freud widened the concept of the transference to include fantasies, as well as memories, directed towards the analyst. Susan Isaacs[2] introduced the term phantasy to distinguish unconscious from conscious fantasy but it has never come into general use, perhaps because there is no rigid barrier between conscious and unconscious, especially in young children.

It has gradually become clear that the hallmark of psychoanalysis is the study of patients' transferred experiences, coupled with the verbal expression to the patient of what has been understood by the analyst. The specific linking of the present response, to the analyst, with past fantasies and memories is called a 'transference interpretation'. There are multitudes of therapists and therapies aiming to relieve people suffering from mental conflict. Some therapists get called, or call themselves, analysts. But unless they focus their attention upon the processes of the transference their techniques are not the same as those of psychoanalysis and therefore their results are not comparable.

A common criticism is that Freud in particular, and psychoanalysts in general, ignored outward reality in their concentration upon studying the inner, unconscious fantasysing aspect of the mind. Schreber[3] was a distinguished German lawyer of the last century who wrote and published an account of his sufferings and elations when he was a patient in a mental hospital. Freud[4] was not consulted by Schreber but became interested in his document, approaching it in search of clues as to the origins of Schreber's, and similar, disturbances. Writing 60 years ago he took the view that Schreber's fears and elations had previously been alive in his unconscious mind but had become unmanageably, and apparently spontaneously, conscious. Freud concluded that Schreber's father had been the original subject of many of these experiences. Obviously many of them were fantasies or had a fantastic component. It could not have been simply a memory of purely physical events which led Schreber to believe, as he did at the height of his distress, that his stomach or genitalia had disappeared. Schreber never acknowledged even the possibility that any of his adult anguish could have been a re-experiencing of childhood responses to parental cruelty nor did he consciously recall his father's method of upbringing. However in his book *Soul Murder* Morton Schatzman[5] describes aspects of Schreber's childhood which were not known to Freud, or consciously to Schreber himself. Schreber senior was a paediatrician consumed with a determination to root out from all children, including his own, their curiosity and questioning, all signs of originality or rebellion. He believed these were the 'bad' aspects of children and thus of human nature. Therefore he felt justified in using not only parental psychological domination but even mechanical physical restraints, such as the one which pulled the child's hair if it dared to bend or turn its head. Many of the pains and torments which Schreber experienced in adult life, without physical cause, were similar to those he must have endured at the hands of his extraordinary father.

In addition to his criticism of Freud's approach Schatzman does include the following quotations:

It remains for the future to decide whether there is more delusion in my theory than I should like to admit, or whether there is more truth in Schreber's than other people are as yet prepared to believe. (Freud[6])

Anyone who was more daring than I am in making interpretations, or who was in touch with Schreber's family and consequently better acquainted with the society in which he moved and with the small events of his life, would find it an easy matter to trace back innumerable details of his delusions to their sources and so discover their meaning . . . (Freud[7])

That the reviewers almost unanimously ignored Schatzman's appreciation of what Freud *did* see is an indication of how much active hostility there still is to the possibility that Freud could ever have been right in any of his observations or conclusions. As early as 1909 Freud[8] commented 'when we cannot understand something we always fall back on abuse'. He also once said, protesting mildly at the obloquy which was his lot, that he had not personally created the unconscious but had merely hit upon a way of studying it.

Freud was concerned with investigating that aspect of the individual mind which had previously been ignored by all but the poets. In the course of a prodigious amount of work he opened the way to further study of many fundamental problems, among them the relationship between memory and fantasy in the developing human being. He himself saw that a logical extension of his work on the continuing influences of childhood experiences in adult life, would be the psychoanalytic study of children themselves. At first he thought that children's emotional problems could only be treated indirectly, through their parents. In his one personal experience of child analysis, which was clinically successful, he used this method. His advice was sought, by a former adult patient and her husband, about their $4\frac{3}{4}$-year-old son because the little fellow had developed such an acute terror of horses that he was unwilling, and at times unable, to go out of the house. Freud encouraged Hans' father to allow the child freedom to talk about his feelings and to write down the discussions so that Freud could advise the father on what to say to the child. Freud's account of the work[8] makes very interesting reading to this day. Indeed this is true of almost all that Freud wrote, even though some of his theories have of course been modified or superseded, often by himself. In 1909 Freud thought that no-one but a father 'could possibly have prevailed on the child to make any such avowals'. Freud gradually changed this opinion.

Then in 1926 Melanie Klein[9] began to give her child patients small toys, pencils and paper, string, etc., to assist them in revealing what was going on in their minds. She found that children used these materials in a way which is exactly comparable to that in which adults reveal their unconscious as well as their conscious feelings by 'free association', that is by saying whatever comes into their minds. Children's activities in the privacy and confidentiality of the consulting-room were also found to be comprehensible in the way that dreams are. So further unknown areas of the child mind became accessible for study.

There are very few parents who can tolerate having their off-spring's most intense feelings revealed to them. Parents are normally most distressed by their own children's suffering. Many of a child's emotional experiences are originally bound to be about its own parents, since they are among the few people with whom a young child has contact. With reference to little Hans Freud wrote 'a neurosis never says foolish things, any more than a dream'. Parents, like any human beings, may find it too hard to see the impact of their behaviour on those they love most. A failure to recognise what one cannot bear to perceive is a well-known human defence mechanism. Investigation of the various manifestations of this defence was begun by Freud, though he was not the first to perceive it.

There is another aspect of the problem of who should help children overcome their fears. The young are very dependent on their parents. Melanie Klein first studied how the child's most intense and often most irrational feelings lead it to be uncertain as to whether what it is experiencing is fact or fantasy. Therefore most children cannot endure their fears of permanently losing their real parents nor their parent's expected recrimination, revenge or reproach when fierce fantasies are revealed to them. A child's capacity to express its feelings can also be powerfully inhibited by mental pain caused by the contrast between its love for the real, concerned parents and its own fantastic views of them. In addition these incomprehensible contrasts can be spontaneously experienced as mental breakdown, as madness, even by very young children. Yet little Hans did talk freely to his father about his fears, feelings and fantasies. And Hans' father had much wider limits of tolerance than most parents can achieve, even today. He listened and recorded, thought about, and consulted Freud about, his small son's mental experiences. Although there were unhelpful and con-fusing aspects of Hans parents' behaviour which they could not change, little Hans' terrors did, as Freud wrote, 'direct his parents attention to the unavoidable difficulties by which a child is confronted when, in the course of his cultural training, he is called upon to overcome the innate instinctual components of his mind'.[10]

Little Hans' mother had previously been helped by Freud and, though the child did not consciously know this, the fact of it obviously played a part in producing a family attitude of trust. Nevertheless it was not until Hans saw with his own eyes that Freud did exist in reality, and not just in his father's imagination, that he made significant progress and became much more readily able to describe contradictory and unrealisable wishes. In Freud's words 'the little patient summoned up courage to describe the details of his phobia . . . and take an active share in the analysis.'[11] He went 'forging ahead' and 'the material brought up . . . far outstripped our powers of understanding.'[12]

Hans knew that Freud, called 'the Professor' in the family, was working to try to understand his fears. On one occasion Hans and his father were discussing the boys' complex feelings towards his baby sister.[13] He had feared that his mother would drop Hanna in the bath and kill her. But as they talked Hans contributed that he himself had really wanted Hanna to die, 'because she screams so'. His father said 'and then you'd be alone with Mummy. A good boy doesn't wish that sort of thing, though.' Hans, not yet 5, 'But he may THINK it.' Father, 'But that isn't good.' Hans, 'If he thinks it, it is good all the same, because you can write it to the Professor.' This exchange reminds me of another such occasion in my own work when I kept a 5-year-old patient waiting some minutes for

her session. She expressed fury both in her face and in her movements as she flounced upstairs and stamped into the consulting-
room. Once there she seized a mug and drank several mugs full of
water. I commented that she was showing how angry and starved
she felt by me keeping her waiting. Lottie promptly replied, 'Well,
you see, I'm thirsty of the truth.'

Both children, Hans and Lottie, 60 years apart in time, support
Freud's view that 'children are more inclined to a love of truth than
are their elders'. He did not mean to imply that adults do not love
the truth, but that they are at times unable to welcome or recognise
unpleasant truths about themselves even though such recognition
may bring relief and an appreciation of the beauty that lies in the
truth of a pattern perceived.

Hans once laughed at an explanation of his father's about where
chickens come from, a much needed preliminary to telling Hans
how babies are made and born. When asked why he laughed Hans
answered, 'Because I like what you've told me.' In the context it is
clear that his laughter was an expression of delighted relief at the
realisation of a truth. At times he responded in a similar way to
truths about himself. The relative ease with which Hans accepted
self-awareness increased Freud's interest in the forces of opposition
to understanding in his adult patients.

In the clinical situation I have described, when my young patient
said she was 'thirsty of the truth' I proceeded to say that I thought
she was also showing me something of how she had felt as a baby,
when waiting for someone she wanted. In other words I went on to
make a 'transference interpretation' to her, drawing a connection
between our relationship and previous ones of a dependent nature.

The detailed working out of who I represented at any time, and
whether indeed I was right at all, involved me and my little patient
in a great deal of work. As Freud had observed of Hans, through
the father's written account, the same wishes were constantly
reappearing. 'The monotony only attaches to the analyst's interpretations of these wishes. For Hans they were not more repetitions
but steps in a progressive development from timid hinting to fully
conscious, undistorted perspicuity.'[14] So, too, with Lottie, I
worked in psychoanalytic psychotherapy with her for several years
after she had been sent to me as a last resort, dangerously ill with
asthma. In the course of Lottie's treatment the symbolic aspect of
personal relationships came to be seen more completely and

consistently by her. At the time she showed her awareness of the truth, or an attempt to understand it, as a source of gratification, Lottie had already had over two years treatment. Under the provocation of waiting she represented my concern by a material substance. In this way she showed, among other things, how mental activity is in constant flux with superseded attitudes remaining alive in the unconscious, available for re-experiencing and re-presentation.

The application of the psychoanalytic technique to the study of the minds of even very young children, as developed by Melanie Klein, seems to me to follow in a logical sequence from Freud's approach to the child which he found still alive in every adult patient. Nor do I see any incompatibility between Freud's[15] theory of the infant's struggle to comprehend its first evidence of external reality, that is of the mother and of her feeding breast, and the modes of mental functioning that the work of Melenie Klein, and of colleagues using her technique, have revealed. As early as 1909 Freud realised that underlying the act of fellatio was probably a mixture of memories and fantasies of sucking at the breast. His advice then to his non-analytic readers still holds good today, it was and is equally applicable to his psychoanalytically trained readers. 'Do not try to understand everthing at once but give a kind of unbiassed attention to every point that arises and await further developments.'

Among those who have worked to develop the field of child psychoanalysis Melanie Klein[9] and Anna Freud[17] have been the most important. The extent to which the concept of transference is applicable to the study of children was a serious cause of disagreement between them. I have already stated my view that concentration upon the various manifestations of the transference is one of the hallmarks of psychoanalysis. Basically the same technique as that used in adults was applied to children by Melanie Klein and still is by those who follow her reasoning, including this writer. It follows that I consider the findings obtained by using this technique with children are as valid as those from the psychoanalysis of adults. Both Donald Winnicott and Michael Fordham (a Jungian analytical psychologist) have used Kleinian technique in their work with children, although not feeling it necessary or desirable to be consistent and apply it to their work with adult patients. In my opinion the evidence of physical and psychological continuity, from the cradle to the grave, is overwhelming. Using a basically similar technique for studying the emotional vicissitudes of humans of all ages is obviously one way of eliminating a variable factor in an extremely complex task.

There is no doubt that much of the professional and lay criticism of Melanie Klein's approach to children, and adults, has been for reasons similar to those which caused so much hostility to Freud's work. Studying even very young children she discovered that they suffer a great deal more conscious and unconscious anxiety than many adults are willing or able to believe. Furthermore she found that much of children's anxiety has its roots in the aggressive components of the child's imaginative life and in its struggle to reconcile its loving and aggressive feelings. Melanie Klein was the first person to psychoanalyse very young children. She was, therefore, the first of many to be surprised at, and at times distressed by, the intensity of little children's suffering, the details of their aggressive fantasies and the inescapable implication that the supposedly infant mind is a hive of activity which is at times violent or painful, or both. Psychoanalysing young children has a powerful emotional impact on the observing analyst, to an extent which makes slow recruitment to this specialty a cause for concern and involves child analysts in a continuing struggle against their own impulses to inhibit the patient rather than enable him to release more and more emotional experience for study.

A 5-year-old boy, Karl, came to me for his first psychotherapy session, stood looking into the drawer of toys and materials provided for him and then said despondently 'You haven't got enough *wild* animals for *me*.' He was expressing his fear that I would not be able to perceive or tolerate the full extent of his aggressive impulses. His despondency seemed a clear expression of disappointment, he had hoped for help with what he unconsciously knew was a problem connected with his hostility.

Karl suffered, in fact, from fits for which no organic cause was found. Unfortunately he could only be seen once weekly. This did not give us enough time to work together and was for him provocative of a great deal of frustration. The analytic technique of tolerant observation, assessing the relationship between events in the session and previous life experiences of the child, putting one's views into words the patient can grasp, is essentially the same in analytical child psychotherapy as in psychoanalysis. But in child psychotherapy, particularly as available now in the National Health Service, the patient is only seen between one and three times weekly. When a patient attends every week-day, as in full psycho-analysis, there is obviously more time for studying the manifestations of the problem. Also it has been found that with a short and regular interval between sessions the patient is very much less tempted to resort to renewed attempts to rid himself of mental conflict in pathological ways.

My young patient was right in his own assessment of the roots of his problem. He had very dominating, greedy and destructive aspects of his nature. He was also extremely sensitive to the pains of self-awareness, so that a comment on a manifestation of his aggressive fantasy life might provoke angry denial, or an anguished fear of never being any good, or terror of being punished for his badness. On one occasion Karl had shown his wish to dominate me by moving all the furniture around. Then he embarked on a search for hidden treasure, talking as he did so. He chose a spot in the wall between two chairs in which he said animals were being fed. He decided a chopper was necessary to open the treasure trove and began enacting the movements required for a break in. I drew the parallel between the room, and myself, with his mother's body and his wish to control and possess its contents by violent means. Karl fell to the floor unconscious, only his arms jerking in vigorous chopping movements with his hands clasped as though gripping a chopper.

The first sign of abnormality which Karl's parents had noted was convulsive twitchings of the hands. Thorough physical investigation did not show any organic disease yet attacks of unconsciousness began to occur. When Karl was brought by his mother to see me for a diagnostic interview she also brought her smaller son. At one point in this first consultation the mother was talking to me while the children made use of the play materials provided. Karl, a very small 5, went up behind his tinier brother who sat playing at a table and made as though to grip him round the neck. But both hands started to twitch involuntarily, which rendered Karl anxiously unable to carry out his obvious intention and also had the effect of drawing his mother's attention away from me. Unfortunately full psychoanalysis was not available for this child and once weekly psychotherapy did not enable him to recover. But in many, many sessions of studying him Karl showed me a great deal which I went on trying to help him see for himself. He did in fact make much progress until adolescence supervened, inevitably arousing even more intense emotions. In the example I have just given Karl was probably consciously aware of his hatred of his little brother. Certainly this was so on many occasions when we were working alone together. Karl tried to deal with the pain of his conflicting feelings by remaining unconscious of his love for his little brother. Furthermore it emerged that he was struggling with the problem of his strong and, to him, incompatible feelings toward his mother, as my first example of a fit during psychotherapy with him showed. One method Karl made use of was to concentrate his affection and appreciation on his mother, keeping his brother as the object of his hostility.

In this short chapter it is not possible to go into details of the complexity and intensity of this boy's emotional life nor of the various family difficulties, including his mother's fear that Karl had an inoperable brain lesion. The work that was done with her revealed that this unusually persistent anxiety concealed considerable hostility to Karl. This mother, too, had difficulty in accepting the evidence of her own mixed feelings. After several years treatment, when Karl at the age of nine was having no fits, boarding school was advised as an attempt to relieve the mutual provocation and lack of understanding in the family, especially between Karl and his mother. This worked well for a while, confirming our assessment of the role of the external 'real' world, in Karl's problems. But he relapsed in adolescence and the prognosis is not at all good.

Melanie Klein[18] has written a detailed account of what took place in the psychoanalysis of an eleven-year-old boy. That patient, Richard, spontaneously called the analytic investigation 'the work' and despite its difficulty was deeply committed to it. Even my much less courageous and younger patient was nearly always eager to attend for his sessions. Much of the difficulty lay in the intensity of his desires and the small amount of time available. Both patients confirmed Susan Isaacs'[2] view that unconscious fantasy (phantasy) is the mental component of instinct, in other words that all urges and desires have a fantasy accompaniment. One conclusion that follows from this important concept is that the mind is in constant activity, always trying to reconcile its perceptions of external reality with the underlying fantasies. In psychoanalytic work with young children the power of fantasy is most vividly revealed. If a person believes that imagining the destruction of the world with urine and flatus can really achieve this aim his bodily functions and ability to play noisily with water are both likely to be affected. That such fears can and do affect children, even normal ones, seems to me beyond doubt. But of course their pleasures can be equally intense and seemingly timeless.

Children do not only fear being attacked or punished, they can also suffer acute anxiety on behalf of the people they love but to whom they have also had hostile impulses. A three-year-old girl in treatment with me for faecal retention once dared to play with water after we had worked for months studying her fears of it. Unfortunately there was a thunderstorm with torrential rain on the way home. The following session the patient was unable even to go near the side of the room where the sink was. As I began to describe her apparent fear she burst out 'Well you see what happened to me yesterday, I nearly got dead, and are you alright? I thought you'd be blown up and drowned too'.

This example shows the way in which it has been found that the analyst's room also represents the analyst and thus fantasies about it have to be studied as an aspect of the transference. The child's fear of me and her fear for me were intense and almost concomitant.

The behaviour and feelings of the real parents are an essential and continuing aspect of the child's world. No child exists or can survive without some communication between its inner world of fantasy and the outer world on which it depends. Physical and emotional growth depend upon their interaction. Smirnoff[19] believes, as do many others, that 'Kleinians thus regard phantasy as the basic ingredient of all mental life'. In my opinion we think we have evidence that phantasy is *one* of the bases of mental life. It is a misunderstanding to suppose that Kleinians systematically and as a group underestimate the equally important mental function of perceiving and learning from external reality. Inevitably what is taken in, physically or psychologically, is affected by fantasy. Part of the common difficulty in accepting this is that fantasy, the unknown, tends to be thought of as destructive. Whereas in fact there are many aspects of fantasy life which enable children to get more out of the environment, and to give more to it, than is offered to them. This important factor in the development of human individuality is related to the problem of the intractable nature of some difficulties affecting people whose families have been of the kind so vividly described by Laing and Esterson.[20] It is simply not true that removing even very young people from a provocative and confusing environment always leads to spontaneous recovery. No more regularly true is the implication that parent substitutes will be unprovocative and comprehensible in their handling of the child or parent.

The most promising recent developments in the psychoanalytic investigation of anxiety, and its impact on the development of mind and personality, have been stimulated by Bion.[21] He took up Melanie Klein's concept of projective identification,[9] a term she used to describe a state in which a part of the self is experienced as expelled into, and to have become part of, the source of gratification or frustration. Bion found this theory to be of great value in understanding adults' psychotic disorders, and their development. He also discovered that projective identification is normally used as a method of communication and learning, predominantly in babies but to some extent throughout life. In early infancy emotional responses are felt to be concrete and as such are projected into the care-taking adult who responds with what Bion calls 'reverie' and in effect translates the baby's experience into abstract concepts about which she can think, act on, forget, dream of, in fact use in ways normally associated with mental activity.

By identifying with this maternal function to perform what Bion calls 'alpha function' the infant begins to develop a capacity to think and feel abstractly. For the baby to respond in this way, which is necessary for normal mental growth, it has to be cared for mainly by one person. This person is still usually the mother, whose role in the foundations of mental health cannot be over-estimated. It is not essential that the baby's main care-taker be its own mother, but there is no doubt that continuity and predictability of care are of fundamental importance to mental health and growth. Bion held the view that the mother, or main care-taker, must not only love the baby but also the baby's father if the function of 'reverie' is to be performed optimally. The implications for babies growing up in unhappy or single-parent homes, as well as in institutions, are manifold and beyond the scope of this article.

I would like to end this contribution by drawing attention to the way in which the increasingly fashionable observational studies of infants, too many to be quoted individually, are providing growing support for the psychoanalysts' point of view that infantile emotional experiences are subtle, important and profoundly relevant to mental health and development in later life.

## Notes

1. Freud, Sigmund, *Fragment of the Analysis of a Case of Hysteria (Dora)*, Standard Edition — vol. VIII (Hogarth, London, 1905).

2. Isaacs, Susan, 'The Nature and Function of Phantasy' in *Developments in Psycho-Analysis* (Hogarth Press, London, 1943).

3. Schreber, F. P., *Den Wurdigkeiten Eirres Nervenkranken* (Leipsig, 1903), Translation, by MacAlpine and Hunter, Memoirs of My Nervous Illness (Dawsons, London, 1955).

4. Freud, Sigmund, *The Case of Schreber*. First published 1911. Translated in the Standard Edition of the Works of Freud (Hogarth Press, London, 1958), p. 78.

5. Schatzman, Morton, *Soul Murder* (Allen Lane, London, 1973), p. 93.

6. Freud, Sigmund, *The Case of Schreber*. First published 1911. Translated in the Standard Edition of the Works of Freud (Hogarth Press, Lodnon, 1958), p. 79.

7. Freud, Sigmund, ibid., p. 57.

8. Freud, Sigmund, *Little Hans* 1909. Standard Edition — vol. X, (Hogarth Press, London, 1955), p. 102.

9. Klein, Melanie, *The Psycho-Analysis of Children* (Hogarth Press, London, 1932).

10. Freud, Sigmund, *Little Hans*, p. 143.

11. Freud, Sigmund, ibid., p. 123.

12. Freud, Sigmund, ibid., p. 127.

13. Freud, Sigmund, ibid., p. 72.

14. Freud, Sigmund, ibid., p. 130.

15. Freud, Sigmund, *Civilization and Its Discontents*. Standard Edition — vol. XXI (Hogarth Press, London, 1930), p. 124.

16. Freud, Sigmund, *Little Hans*, p. 7.

17. Freud, Anna, *The Psycho-Analytical Treatment of Children* (Hogarth Press, London, 1964).

18. Klein, Melanie, *The Narrative of a Child Analysis* (Hogarth Press, London, 1961).

19. Smirnoff, Victor, *The Scope of Child Analysis* 1966. (Translation published by Routledge and Kegan Paul, London, 1971), p. 160.

20. Laing, R. D. and Esterson, A., *Sanity, Madness and The Family* (Tavistock Publications, London, 1964).

21. Bion, Wilfred R., *Learning from Experience* (Heineman, London, 1962).

# 2 RECOGNITION AND MONITORING OF ANXIETY BY MEANS OF PSYCHOMETRIC TESTS

David Jones

## Introduction

The assessment of anxiety is a problem of direct concern to everyone involved in attempts to classify the personality characteristics of children as well as those involved in the interpretation of the results of psychometric tests administered to school children for the purposes of estimating their intellectual potential and academic achievement levels. The problem is the exceedingly difficult one of isolating a complex personality characteristic so that inferences may be made about its possible effects on the child's intellectual functioning, school performance and his or her relationships with adults and other children. While there is universal agreement on the importance of anxiety there is less of a general consensus on the exact nature of the concept. Different workers have reported attempts to measure such constructs as manifest anxiety, general anxiety, test anxiety, state anxiety, trait anxiety, social anxiety, emotionality, neuroticism, fear, separation anxiety, moral anxiety, adjustment and stability. There are important theoretical distinctions between some of these constructs. One of the most important general distinctions from the point of view of definition and interpretation of findings, is the dichotomy which has been emphasised by Cattell and Scheier[1] and by Spielberger[2] between state-anxiety and trait-anxiety. State-anxiety is a transitory reaction to stress consisting of unpleasant subjective feelings of tension and apprehension and associated autonomic nervous system activity. In contrast trait-anxiety is a relatively stable personality characteristic and refers to individual differences in anxiety proneness. Clearly these two constructs are related and the likelihood of a child experiencing state-anxiety will be determined in part by the level of trait-anxiety. Children with high levels of trait-anxiety will be more prone than other children to experience state-anxiety in stressful situations and they may well find more situations to be stressful.

Traditionally psychometric tests have been categorised according to the procedure involved as either projective or non-projective. A separate chapter in this book discusses applications of projective measures of anxiety so they will not be considered any further here. Broadly speaking non-projective tests of anxiety can be split into four general groups. (a) Questionnaires or inventories requiring direct responses by the children. (b) Rating scales of children's behaviour completed by the parents, teachers, classmates or others who have been in contact with them. (c) Objective tests which are not in themselves direct measures of anxiety. (d) Physiological techniques for measuring arousal and autonomic reactivity. By far the largest number of tests of anxiety in children fall into the category of direct questionnaires. The objective test category is perhaps more arbitrary than the others. It will be used in this chapter to include some discussion of the practice of inferring anxiety levels from consideration of test profiles in intellectual assessments.

It must be stated at the outset that there are considerable doubts about the validity of any single method for the measurement of anxiety in children and that where decisions have to be made regarding the future of the individual child it is advisable to obtain as wide as possible a range of measures coming from several of these different approaches. At the present stage of development the various measures of anxiety are far from interchangeable. It will be seen that many of the measures of anxiety were developed in the first instance as research instruments intended for use with groups of subjects. While these tests provide extremely important methods for estimating the effects of anxiety level on behaviour and performance, it is an abuse of their function to apply them as isolated measures of anxiety in a clinical investigation.

There is a vast literature on the development and use of the various methods of measuring anxiety in children and reviews by Ruebush,[3] Sarason,[4] McReynolds[5] and Gaudry and Spielberger[6] provide summaries of the early literature.

## Questionnaire Methods

The majority of questionnaire methods in current use as measures of anxiety in children have been derived from similar instruments which were developed earlier to measure anxiety levels in adults. It follows that the theoretical bases for the techniques are those advanced in support of the adult instruments. This practice at least permits attempts at direct comparison of anxiety levels in adults and children and is beginning to provide some insight into long-term developmental changes in anxiety levels.

In general questionnaires and inventories consist of a series of items each of which describes a way the child may feel about himself or herself, about interactions with others or about the surroundings. In most cases the subject is required to respond by indicating agreement or disagreement with the statement made in each item, although in some cases a gradation of the response may be necessary. The standard practice in questionnaire construction is to attempt to control for response bias and other unwanted tendencies by wording the items so that loading on the scale is given for agreement on some items and disagreement on others. Unfortunately on a number of the anxiety scales for children either because of practical difficulties in the wording of the items or following the individual test constructor's preference this practice has not been accepted. Typically one or more points are allocated for each anxiety response on the questionnaire and scoring is cumulative resulting in a total anxiety score for the scale.

Questionnaires have the great advantage that they can be administered to groups of subjects simultaneously. In cases where the subjects are required to read the questions silently to themselves and then respond the burden is on the examiner to determine that the children and also adolescents have adequate reading ability to understand the items. General instructions to ask for help when confronted by difficult words may be inadequate particularly in the case of anxious children. For some scales the standard practice is for the examiner to read out the items and adequate cooperation from all members of the group is necessary.

Many anxiety questionnaires are administered together with a lie scale. In most cases the original intention of the selected lie scale was to provide a measure of the tendency of the subject to fake responses. The lie scale items generally represent highly desirable behavioural characteristics or fears and anxieties that most people possess. While the possession of some of these characteristics and the denial of some of the fears is perfectly acceptable, too high a score on the lie scale may indicate dishonesty, defensiveness or just lack of cooperation. A high score on the lie scale indicates that the score of that child on the anxiety scale and scores on other personality dimensions must be treated with considerable caution. A number of studies have found the scores on the various lie scales to be interesting in themselves. For example, Eysenck[7] has reported that lie scores decline with increasing age in children and she suggests that they may provide a measure of social maturity.

Since by far the greatest amount of work on the assessment of anxiety in children has involved the use of questionnaire techniques some of the better known instruments and also a few of the less well known ones will be described briefly on the following pages.

### The Children's Manifest Anxiety Scales (CMAS)

The Taylor Manifest Anxiety Scale (MAS) which is the adult version of the CMAS consists of 50 statements such as, 'I worry more than other people', selected from the MMPI on the basis of the judgements of a group of clinical psychologists to be indicative of manifest anxiety.[8] Although descriptive of clinical state the MAS was intended to provide a measure related to drive in the Hullian learning theory sense. The CMAS consists of 42 items selected from the MAS and modified to make them more suitable for use with children.[9] Examples of the items are: 'I have trouble swallowing' and 'I worry when I go to bed at night'. The anxiety score is obtained by summing all the 'Yes' responses. The CMAS also contains an 11-item lie scale containing items like 'I tell the truth every single time'.

Much of the research work involving the CMAS, as also in the case of the MAS, has been involved in testing predictions generated from Hull-Spence Learning Theory on the relations between drive level and performance. In particular there have been a number of attempts to test the prediction that high-anxiety subjects perform better than low-anxiety subjects on simple tasks, but that they perform less well than low-anxiety subjects on complex tasks in which competing incorrect responses have high 'habit strengths'. As a test the CMAS is a measure of the tendency to experience anxiety rather than the transitory experience and it can be considered as a measure of trait-anxiety.

The original standardisation group for the scale consisted of American 4th to 6th Grade children, but it has been used with somewhat younger groups. For older children the tendency is to use the MAS. The scale is relatively easy to administer and score and the test-retest reliability is adequate. A short form of the CMAS has been devised,[10] and the use of 'verbal' and 'somatic' subscales has been suggested.[11]

*The Test Anxiety Scale for Children (TASC)*

This scale is derived from an earlier adult version, the Test Anxiety Questionnaire (TAQ) which was devised by Mandler and Sarason[12] to measure the anxiety reactions of adults to examinations and tests. The TASC has been developed and used extensively by Sarason and his associates[13,14] as a means of measuring the anxiety aroused in children by tests and classroom situations. Behind the construction of the test is the psychoanalytic view expressed by Sarason that the anxiety reaction of the test anxious child is determined by earlier life experiences in the home. In particular earlier experiences of having behaviour evaluated by parents and other adults is likely to affect the child's reactions to test-like situations. The TASC consists of 30 questions, such as 'When the teacher says that she is going to find out how much you have learned, does your heart begin to beat faster?' The items all refer to some aspect of test or classroom situations. The questions are always read to the class and the children are not required to read them themselves, the score being the number of times the child enters 'Yes' on the answer sheet. Test-retest reliability for the scale is adequate and there is some evidence of a positive relation between ratings by class teachers of anxiety and TASC scores.

An important feature of Sarason's theory is that it predicts a negative correlation between TASC scores and academic achievement and numerous studies have been carried out to test this hypothesis. Hill and Sarason in a longitudinal study in the United States found that negative correlation between TASC scores and test performance continued to increase in magnitude throughout the elementary school period.[14] They also suggest that anxiety is more closely related to reading than to arithmetic in the early years at school, but that the difference weakens and disappears later. In general the balance of evidence seems to support the prediction of a low negative correlation between test anxiety and academic attainment, but the pattern of results for reading and arithmetic has not always been obtained by other workers. For example, Cox working with 4th and 5th Grade Australian children found that TASC scores were negatively correlated with arithmetic, but they were not correlated with reading scores.[15] An earlier study by Lynn using a different anxiety measure also indicated that there was a tendency for anxious pupils to do better at reading than at arithmetic.[16] It seems that the pattern of emphasis placed on different subjects at school is likely to affect the relation.

## The General Anxiety Scale for Children (GASC)

The GASC was constructed by Sarason and his associates at Yale University to provide a measure of general anxiety which has the same format and is administered in the same way as the TASC.[13] Examples of questions in the general scale are: 'If you were to climb a ladder, would you worry about falling off it?', and 'Do you think you worry more than other boys and girls?'. The test has adequate test-retest reliability, although it has been observed that mean scores on a second administration tend to be slightly lower than on first administration. As a measure of general anxiety the scale has been less widely used than the CMAS.

Embedded within the GASC is an 11-item lie scale referred to as the Lie Scale for Children (LSC). All of the items contain the word *ever*, examples of the questions being: 'Has anyone ever been able to scare you?' and 'Are you ever unhappy?'. The lie scale is specifically designed as a measure of the tendency to deny feelings of anxiety and not as a general measure of defensiveness. A further scale developed for use with the TASC and GASC is the Defensiveness Scale for Children (DSC). The DSC is made up of the GASC Lie Scale together with items intended to detect the tendency to deny negative feelings, e.g. 'Are there some people that you don't like?' Variations in the form and scoring of defensiveness scales have been used in a number of studies.

## The IPAT Scales

The work of Cattell and his associates at the Institute for Personality and Ability Testing (IPAT) at Illinois has produced a series of questionnaires for the measurement of personality characteristics. Probably the best known is the 16PF which measures 15 personality dimensions and intelligence in adults. One adaptation is the Children's Personality Questionnaire (CPQ)[17] designed for children aged 8 to 12 years. The CPQ yields scores on 14 dimensions, one of which is a measure of intelligence. The 14 primary source traits, as Cattell refers to them, were derived by factor analytic techniques. By intercorrelating and factoring the primary source traits it is possible to obtain scores on the two higher order factors of anxiety and extraversion. The scores on 6 of the primary traits are used in the equation to calculate the anxiety score. These traits are D (Phlegmatic vs. Excitable), O (Self-assured vs. Apprehensive), Q4 (Relaxed vs. Tense), Q3 (Casual vs. Controlled), C

(Affected by Feelings vs. Emotionally Stable) and H (Shy vs. Venturesome). There are two forms of the test available, Forms A and B, and each form is divided into two parts for ease of administration. Each form can take up to 50 minutes and for clinical use the administration of both forms is recommended. For testing individual children this is a considerable investment in testing time on the part of the examiner and the child. Normally the child is expected ιo read the questions himself, but with instructions to ask for help if he does not understand a word. In contrast to the other questionnaires described above all of the questions in the CPQ are in a forced choice form and the child must choose between two alternatives, e.g. 'Do you have many friends *or* just a few good friends?'

Cattell considers that the scale provides a measure of what he describes as free-floating, manifest anxiety which may be influenced by long-term and situational variables. Considered together with the 16PF and the other scales in this series, the CPQ is an important research instrument for the longitudinal study of personality development. Caution is still necessary in the interpretation of the anxiety score of the individual child.

For younger children there is the Early School Personality Questionnaire (ESPQ).[18] This test is suitable for children aged 6 to 8 years and measures 13 primary source traits. Again it is possible to extract a second-order anxiety factor. The questionnaire is designed for group administration to classes of 20 to 30 children in this younger age group. All of the questions are read aloud to the children who record their responses on record forms that are well-designed and extremely easy to use. As in the CPQ on each item the child must choose between alternative statements. Testing time can take from 60 to 100 minutes and can be spread over two sessions.

The version of the IPAT tests suitable for adolescents is The Junior-Senior High School Personality Questionnaire (HSPQ).[19] Equivalent forms of the test are available, each form taking about 40 to 50 minutes to administer. Scores are obtained on 14 dimensions and again a second-order anxiety factor can be extracted.

When the main concern is the measurement of anxiety it is possible to use one of the separate IPAT Anxiety Scales rather than the multi-factor versions of the questionnaires. The adult version has the title 'Self Analysis Form' on the test booklet.[20] It is made up of 40 items taken from the five primary traits in the 16PF which load on the anxiety factor. This Anxiety Scale is considered suitable for adolescents of 14 years and over as a measure of free-floating, manifest anxiety. More recently the Child Anxiety Scale (CAS) has become available.[21] Taking the criterion of the ESPQ second-order anxiety factor Gillis has constructed a scale of 20 items each of which presents the child with two clear choices. There is an easy to use answer sheet on which each item is identified by a drawing, e.g. a butterfly, a spoon. The instructions and all of the items are read out to the children. A tape-recorded version of the test administration is available and normative data are provided for children in the age range 5 to 12 years. The test-retest reliabilities quoted are quite good. Small groups of children can be tested together in a little over 15 minutes. This is a useful quick screening test for anxiety particularly for primary school children.

*The Maudsley and Eysenck Scales*

The Junior Eysenck Personality Inventory (JEPI) like the Maudsley Personality Inventory (MPI) and the Eysenck Personality Inventory (EPI), the two adult scales from which it is derived, measures the two personality dimensions neuroticism (or emotionality) (N) and extraversion-introversion (E). The test has been developed by S. G. B. Eysenck[7,22] and is intended for use with children in the 7 to 16 years age range. There are British and American forms available. The scale is made up of 60 items selected on the basis of factor analytic studies, 24 to measure the N factor, 24 to measure the E factor and 12 items making up the lie scale. It is possible to draw theoretical distinctions between the constructs of anxiety and neuroticism while accepting that the two are highly correlated.[1] The N scale of the JEPI is included here as a test which can and has been used as an estimate of the anxiety or emotionality level of children. The test has good reliability and separate norms are available for boys and girls. There appears to be an increase in the mean scores for girls over the stated age range but no change for boys.

The New Junior Maudsley Inventory (NJMI) has been developed by Furneaux and Gibson[23] to serve as a form of the MPI suitable for children in the 9 to 16 years age range. The point is made in the manual that the children should have mental and reading ages of at least 9 years and it is recommended that for group use there should be one experienced examiner for each 15 subjects. As in the case of the JEPI described above, the NJMI provides measures on the

Neuroticism and Extraversion dimensions. There are 22 items in each of these scales and 18 items making up a lie scale. An earlier version of the test, the Junior Maudsley Personality Inventory, did not contain the lie scale, although many of the normative data were collected on this version of the test. The NJMI can be regarded as an alternative to the JEPI for a slightly narrower age range of children. A discussion of some of the major findings on the use of both scales is provided by Rachman.[24]

A more recent development is the Junior version of the Eysenck Personality Questionnaire (EPQ).[25] This test is similar in many respects to the JEPI, but in addition to the E, N and Lie Scales it has the P factor which is a measure of psychoticism. Normative data are available for children in the age range 7 to 15 years. However, test-retest reliabilities for the younger ages are rather low. For 10 years of age and older the reliabilities are quite high. Girls again show an increase in mean N scores as a function of increasing age whereas the means for boys are relatively stable across the age range.

### The State-Trait Anxiety Inventory For Children (STAIC)

The STAIC was developed from the State-Trait Anxiety Inventory (STAI) which was constructed by Spielberger and his associates[26] to provide measures of anxiety for adolescents and adults. The STAIC[27] consists of two separate self-report scales, one to measure state anxiety (A-State) and the other to measure trait anxiety (A-Trait). The A-State scale contains 20 statements which ask children how they feel at the time they are actually taking the test. For each statement there is a choice of three boxes and the child must select one, e.g. the choice between: I feel . . . . . 'very frightened', 'frightened' and 'not frightened'. For half of the items the 'very' term indicates the presence of anxiety and for the other items it indicates the absence of anxiety, as in 'very satisfied'. The A-Trait scale contains 20 statements which the children must respond to in terms of how they generally feel. For example: I feel unhappy . . . . . 'hardly ever', 'sometimes' and 'often'. The 'often' response is given the highest anxiety weighting for all of the A-Trait items. The STAIC is intended for use with children in the age range 9 years to 12 years and for younger children with at least average reading ability. Older subjects can be given the STAI. Since the A-State scale is designed to measure transitory anxiety states it is potentially suitable for repeated use on different occasions to monitor reactions to stress, changes experienced during psycho-therapy or as a measure of the effectiveness of desensitisation during behaviour therapy. Both scales can usually be administered in about 20 minutes and subjects who have experience of the A-State scale can complete it in about 5 minutes on repeated administrations. Normative data are available for American school children.

### The Achievement Anxiety Test (AAT)

The AAT is a test that is more suitable for use with students, but it can be used with older school children. Devised by Alpert and Haber[28] the test differs in intention from the TASC in that it attempts to measure the facilitating effects of anxiety on examina-tion performance as well as the debilitating effects. The test consists of nine items based on a prototype statement 'Anxiety helps me to do better during examinations and tests' and a 10-item debilitating scale based on a prototype statement 'Anxiety inter-feres with my performance during examinations and tests'. The concept of facilitating anxiety is an interesting one and its role in the academic performance of school children merits further investigation.

### The Multiple Affect Adjective Check List (MAACL)

The MAACL[29,30] provides a good example of the use of adjective check lists in the measurement of anxiety and other personality characteristics. Tests of this sort have been used mainly with adult subjects but the scales are suitable for experimental use with older school children. The MAACL consists of 132 adjectives arranged in alphabetical order in each of two forms. In the 'In General' form the subject is required to mark the words which describe 'How you generally feel' and in the 'Today' form to mark the words describing 'How you feel now — today'. The test yields three scores: anxiety, depression and hostility. It is easy to administer and has been widely used as a research instrument. Nevertheless, the clinical validity of these measures remains to be demonstrated convincingly.

### The Jesness Inventory

This is a self-report inventory devised by Jesness to provide a means for distinguishing between delinquents and non-delinquents and to provide a common basis for the description of some of the personality characteristics of both groups.[31,32] A variety of scores can be obtained, but the one that is of interest here is the measure of social anxiety which is thought to represent emotional discomfort associated with interpersonal relationships.

## The Family Relations Test

This test is sometimes considered as a projective technique but its construction is interesting and in essence it is a forced-choice inventory. Devised by Bene and Anthony[33] the test has different questions for younger children in the age range 3 to 7 years and older children in the range 7 to 15 years. The child selects a series of figures to represent the different members of the family and behind each figure is an attached box. The task is to place a series of statements into the boxes attached to the figures to which the statements best apply. While the test does not directly measure anxiety it provides estimates of the positive and negative feelings that the child has for different members of his family which may be valuable in a clinical situation when taken along with more direct estimates of anxiety.

## Behaviour Rating Scales

Rating scales of this category represent an attempt to standardise and facilitate the way in which one individual assesses or describes the behaviour of another. Of necessity the type of assessment that is possible depends upon the judgement of the person rating the behaviour and his or her relationship with the child concerned. The ratings may be influenced by unwanted contamination of factors such as halo effects, order effects and the characteristics of the rater. At one extreme the ratings are made by trained observers which achieves considerable objectivity and high inter-observer reliability. However, such assessments may be limited by the observer's lack of close familiarity with the child. In the rating of traits such as anxiety the assessments are often made by teachers. Here there is sometimes variability in the familiarity of the teacher with the method and with the children to be assessed. In other situations ratings are made by parents or others who have been in reasonably close contact with the child. At the other extreme from the use of a trained observer is the technique of obtaining ratings from children on the behaviour of their classmates. Sociometric procedures of this sort should not be undertaken lightly, particularly in situations where the children will continue to share the same environment. One of the few advantages of behaviour rating scales over self-report inventories is that the direct coopera- tion of the child being assessed is not necessary. Thus it becomes possible to obtain estimates of typical behaviour even when the child is disturbed or uncooperative at the time of assessment. A few examples are given of rating scales completed by teachers and by parents.

*Rating Scales Completed by Teachers*

One of the most widely used rating scales in the United States for completion by teachers is the Conners Teachers Rating Scale (TRS).[34] It consists of 39 items arranged in three general classes: group participation, classroom behaviour and attitude towards authority. Each item is rated by the teacher from the following four choices — 'not at all', 'just a little', 'pretty much' or 'very much'. Factor analysis of the scale produced five general item clusters: aggressive conduct, daydreaming-inattention, anxiety-fearfulness, hyperactivity and sociability-cooperation.

The Bristol Social Adjustment Guides (BSAG) have been widely used as behaviour checklists to be completed by teachers to provide an index of maladjustment in school settings. Early editions of the BSAG had indicated that a measure of Anxiety for Adult Attention could be obtained. In the Fifth Edition[35] of the BSAG anxiety is no longer maintained as a taxonomic category and it is suggested that in the school situation anxiety is associated with both over-reacting and under-reacting behaviours. Anxiety measures can be obtained from the versions of the Guides for rating the Child in the Family, usually completed by the parent, and the Child in Residential Care, usually completed by a social worker who knows the child well.

The Devereux Behaviour Rating Scales devised by Spivack and his associates cover three different age groups of children and adolescents.[36–38] The ratings take about 15 minutes and are best made by a teacher who has observed the child in the classroom. Scores can be obtained on a number of dimensions such as achieve- ment anxiety and proneness to emotional upset.

*Rating Scales Completed by Parents*

A major problem with rating scales completed by parents is poor test-retest reliability. Also ratings by fathers frequently differ from ratings by mothers. One of the most detailed rating scales is the Personality Inventory for Children (PIC) which amounts to a children's version of the Minnesota Multiphasic Personality Inventory (MMPI) completed by the parents rather than the children. There are 600 items. Anxiety is one of the 14 clinical subscales.[39]

A shorter rating scale is the Conners Parent Symptom Questionnaire (PSQ)[34] which is similar in structure to the Teacher Rating Scale. The revised version consists of 48 items four of which contribute to the score on anxiety. There is also a category called 'Psychosomatic Problems'.

An example of a research instrument which attempts to give a more detailed measure of anxiety from parents' ratings is the Louisville Behavior Check List.[40] Part of the test is an 18 item Fear Scale of which six of the items refer to sleep disturbances and other items refer to fears of the dark and death. There are also measures of unlikeableness and somatic complaints.

## Objective Techniques

The use of objective tests as indicators of anxiety level in adults has attracted a great deal of interest and to a lesser extent some of the procedures have been used at a research level as measures of anxiety in children. In almost all cases the subject is unaware that anxiety is the aspect of behaviour that is being measured by the test. Starting with this assumption it follows that the subject should be less able to fake responses in objective tests than in responding to questionnaires. An extremely wide range of tests have been used in various studies as possible indicators of anxiety, but there has been relatively little in the way of standardisation of procedures between workers and there is a lack of extensive normative data. In the space available it is not possible to do more than mention a few of the types of task that have been studied. Psychomotor tasks such as tapping speed, hand steadiness and two-hand coordination have been used in a number of studies and various verbal learning tasks such as serial learning and paired associated learning have also been considered to be important. Two important papers, one by Stevenson and Odon[41] using children as subjects and one by Martin[42] involving adult subjects, effectively demonstrate the low correlation between different measures of anxiety. Nevertheless on the basis of factor analysis of the results of 98 subjects on a large number of tests that others have used as measures of anxiety Martin identified an anxiety factor which was relatively independent of both intelligence and motivation.

Both Cattell and Eysenck have selected objective tests by factor analytic techniques on the basis of their loadings on a general anxiety factor. The Objective-Analytic (O-A) Anxiety Battery developed by Cattell and Scheier[1] represents one attempt to combine pencil and paper tests and objective measures. The battery is suitable for research use with subjects of 14 years and over.

A final method to be considered in this section is the practice of attempting to infer anxiety levels of children from evaluation of the profiles of subtest scores on individual intelligence test scales. The use of the Wechsler Intelligence Scale for Children-Revised (WISC-R) will be taken as an example. The tester should always be sensitive to any signs of anxiety shown by the child in the test situation. Sometimes shy and withdrawn children have to be gently coaxed into making audible responses. Obtaining accurate estimates of verbal abilities from such children can be difficult and time-consuming. A much more difficult problem to assess is that of the possible effects of anxiety on arousal and attention and the consequential effects on test performance. Evidence from the results of factor analysis of subtest scores of the WISC-R by Kaufman[43,44] suggests the presence of three factors found repeatedly at different age levels. The first two factors are Verbal Comprehension (which was found to have primary loadings on Information, Similarities, Vocabulary and Comprehension) and Perceptual Organization (which was found to have primary loadings on Picture Completion, Picture Arrangement, Block Design, Object Assembly and Mazes). These two factors resemble the traditional Verbal and Performance Scales. The third factor is called Freedom from Distractability and has primary loadings on Arithmetic, Digit Span and Coding. This factor has been interpreted in different ways and for some children it has been suggested that the three subtests Arithmetic, Digit Span and Coding form the 'anxiety triad'. Lutey suggested that it is a measure of freedom from disruptive anxiety.[45] Wechsler in discussing the original Wechsler Bellevue Scale, an intelligence scale for adults, considered that low scores on the Digit Span, Digit Symbol (Coding) and Arithmetic subtests may sometimes be an indication of anxiety.[46] There is considerable support for the notion that one or more of these subtests may be influenced by anxiety, with Digit Span seeming to be the most frequently susceptible. The evidence is that these effects are related more to state-anxiety or test anxiety rather than to trait-anxiety.

## Physiological Techniques

Discussion of the physiology of anxiety is beyond the scope of this chapter. Distinctions between what is meant by arousal and emotional reactivity are often blurred in the literature. Almost certainly the limbic system and the reticular activating system are involved in complex interaction with both the sympathetic and parasympathetic branches of the autonomic nervous system. In addition there is both cortical and sub-cortical involvement. In recent years there has been a marked increase in the use of physiological techniques to measure reactivity of the autonomic nervous system in adults. In addition there has been considerable research activity in the study of such measures as heart rate in newborn infants. In contrast to these two areas of activity little has been done in the way of normative data collection of physiological measures in children of school age. In part this is because much of the work is still of a research nature and some of the procedures are tedious and time-consuming. There is the added difficulty that the complex recording procedures induce anxiety in some children and so may interfere directly with the state they are intended to measure. With the continued improvement of telemetric techniques allowing the subject to be freed from physical restraint by connecting wires it should become far easier to measure some of these variables in children without causing stress and discomfort.

Venables has provided a good recent review of autonomic reactivity in children and also a guide to further discussion of instrumentation.[47,48] The two systems which have been studied in most detail in children have been electrodermal and cardiac activity. Electrodermal measures seem largely to reflect sympathetic nervous system activity whereas cardiac reactivity reflects the balance between sympathetic and parasympathetic activity. Heart rate deceleration may result from increased parasympathetic nervous system activity or decreased sympathetic nervous system activity. A further problem is the range of individual differences in 'response specificity' of physiological variables. Some measures appear to be sensitive to emotional change in some subjects and not in others. Simultaneous recordings from several systems on a polygraph give a better indication of reactivity.

While the majority of studies employing physiological techniques have been concerned with demonstrating the pattern of heightened autonomic responding in anxious subjects, there have been attempts to demonstrate that some deviant groups such as delinquents show less change in autonomic activity than normals exposed to the same stimulation. For example, Davies and Maliphant found that adolescent boys judged by teachers to be refractory had lower base heart rates than controls and that they showed less change in heart rate in response to stress than the controls.[49]

## Concluding Comments

The diversity of the questionnaires, rating scales and other methods for assessing anxiety is in itself an indication that the field is still in a state of development. The problem of definition has been mentioned earlier. In attempting to assess the relation between anxiety and educational attainment it is particularly important to recognise the different aims of the various assessment instruments. Too often it is apparent that the correlations involving general anxiety scales such as the CMAS and narrower scales such as the TASC are quoted and compared indiscriminately. The general conclusion that can be drawn from the large and varied literature is that there appears to be a low negative correlation, often reaching a statistically significant level, between anxiety measures and various aspects of academic achievement. It also seems that the specific measures of test anxiety are a little more likely to show the negative correlation than the general scales. These effects are by no means consistent across all studies and there are differing patterns of correlation for different academic variables. There is an indication that the negative effects of anxiety tend to increase with increasing age over much of the school period. Another general observation is that the mean anxiety scores for groups of girls tend to be slightly higher than the mean anxiety scores for groups of boys of the same age. However, there is some conflict of evidence on the relative disabling effects of anxiety level on academic achievement in boys and girls. Such factors as the sex of the teacher, the method of instruction and the use of differing patterns of discipline for the two sexes may be involved.[50]

It is surprising how few studies have looked for anything more than a linear correlation between anxiety and achievement. There are theoretical grounds for expecting a curvilinear relation if the range of anxiety levels is large. Applying the Yerkes-Dodson law one would expect an inverted U-shape relation between anxiety and performance. The pattern is complicated as the optimum drive or anxiety level for any given task is a function of the task difficulty, and what is difficult for any given subject is determined largely by intelligence level and the amount of practice he or she has had on similar tasks. Thus with heterogeneous groups of subjects and even with many groups of apparently homogeneous subjects concentration on the linear relation between anxiety and some other measure may be misleading. Neglect of the complexity of the relations between different measures is often a weakness in factor analytic studies.

Cattell has put forward the view that the only satisfactory approach to the measurement of anxiety is a multivariate one.[51] Combining a multivariate approach with repeated measures from the same subject it is possible to separate the state and trait components of anxiety. In clinical practice with individual children there is rarely the time for detailed repeated assessments. Inventories can be used to estimate general anxiety proneness. Children who appear to show pathological levels of anxiety on screening require further assessment including the collection of information from parents and teachers. Separate attempts to measure test anxiety and state anxiety should be considered whenever there are suggestions of learning difficulties or behavioural problems at school. On-going monitoring of these measures will provide a useful supplementary index of change as a function of therapy, remedial support or other form of intervention. Usually a short checklist like the STAIC or an adjective checklist together with a couple of short objective performance measures will provide some indication of change. Further work is needed to provide normative data for repeated assessments.

## References

1. Cattell, R. B. and Scheier, I. H., *The Meaning and Measurement of Neuroticism and Anxiety* (Institute for Personality and Ability Testing, Champaign, Illinois, 1961).

2. Spielberger, C. D., 'Theory and Research on Anxiety' in C. D. Spielberger (ed.) *Anxiety and Behavior* (Academic Press, New York, 1966), pp. 3–19.

3. Ruebush, B. K., 'Anxiety' in H. W. Stevenson (ed.) *Child Psychology: The Sixty-second Yearbook of the National Society for the Study of Education* (University of Chicago Press, Chicago, 1963), pp. 460–516.

4. Sarason, S. B., 'The Measurement of Anxiety in Children: Some Questions and Problems' in C. D. Spielberger (ed.) *Anxiety and Behavior* (Academic Press, New York, 1966), pp. 63–79.

5. McReynolds, P., 'The Assessment of Anxiety: a Survey of Available Techniques' in P. McReynolds (ed.) *Advances in Psychological Assessment*, vol. 1 (Science and Behavior Books, Palo Alto, 1968), pp. 244–64.

6. Gaudry, E. and Spielberger, C. D., *Anxiety and Educational Achievement* (Wiley, Sydney, 1971).

7. Eysenck, S. B. G., 'Personality Dimensions in Children' in H. J. Eysenck and S. B. G. Eysenck (ed.) *Personality Structure and Measurement* (Routledge and Kegan Paul, London, 1969), pp. 265–316.

8. Taylor, J. A., 'A Personality Scale of Manifest Anxiety', *Journal of Abnormal and Social Psychology*, **48** (1953), pp. 285–90.

9. Castaneda, A., McCandless, B. R. and Palermo, D. S., 'The Children's Form of the Manifest Anxiety Scale', *Child Development*, **27** (1956), pp. 317–26.

10. Levy, N., 'A Short Form of the Children's Manifest Anxiety Scale', *Child Development*, **29** (1958), pp. 153–4.

11. Reese, H. W., 'Manifest Anxiety and Achievement Test Performance', *Journal of Educational Psychology*, **52** (1961), pp. 132–5.

12. Mandler, G. and Sarason, S. B., 'A Study of Anxiety and Learning', *Journal of Abnormal and Social Psychology*, **47** (1952), pp. 166–73.

13. Sarason, S. B., Davidson, K. S., Lighthall, F. F., Waite, R. R. and Ruebush, B. K., *Anxiety in Elementary School Children* (Wiley, New York, 1960).

14. Hill, K. T. and Sarason, S. B., 'The Relation of Test Anxiety and Defensiveness to Test and School Performance Over the Elementary School Years', *Monographs of the Society for Research in Child Development*, **31**, no. 2 (1966).

15. Cox, F. N., 'Test Anxiety and Achievement Behavior Systems Related to Examination Performance in Children', *Child Development*, **35** (1964), pp. 907–16.

16. Lynn, R., 'Temperamental Characteristics Related to Disparity of Attainment in Reading and Arithmetic', *British Journal of Psychology*, **27** (1957), pp. 62–7.

17. Porter, R. B. and Cattell, R. B., *The Children's Personality Questionnaire* (Institute for Personality and Ability Testing, Champaign, Illinois, 1963).

18. Coan, R. W. and Cattell, R. B., *Early School Personality Questionnaire* (Institute for Personality and Ability Testing, Champaign, Illinois, 1966).

19. Cattell, R. B., *The Junior-Senior High School Personality Questionnaire* (Institute for Personality and Ability Testing, Champaign, Illinois, 1965).

20. Cattell, R. B. and Scheier, I. H., *The IPAT Anxiety Scale* (Institute for Personality and Ability Testing, Champaign, Illinois, 1963).

21. Gillis, J. S., *Child Anxiety Scale Manual* (Institute for Personality and Ability Testing, Champaign, Illinois, 1980).

22. Eysenck, S. B. G., *Manual of the Junior Eysenck Personality Inventory* (University of London Press, London, 1965).

23. Furneaux, W. D. and Gibson, H. B., *The New Junior Maudsley Personality*

*Inventory* (University of London Press, London, 1966).

24. Rachman, S., 'Extraversion and Neuroticism in Childhood' in H. J. Eysenck and S. B. G. Eysenck (eds) *Personality Structure and Measurement* (Routledge and Kegan Paul, London, 1969), pp. 253–64.

25. Eysenck, H. J. and Eysenck, S. B. G., *Manual of the Eysenck Personality Questionnaire* (Hodder and Stoughton, London, 1975).

26. Spielberger, C. D., Gorsuch, R. L. and Lushene, R. E., *Manual for the State-Trait Anxiety Inventory* (Consulting Psychologists Press, Palo Alto, 1970).

27. Spielberger, C. D., Edwards, D. C., Montouri, J. and Lushene, R. E., *The State-Trait Anxiety Inventory for Children* (Consulting Psychologists Press, Palo Alto, 1970).

28. Alpert, R. and Haber, R. N., 'Anxiety in Academic Achievement Situations', *Journal of Abnormal and Social Psychology*, **61** (1960), pp. 207–15.

29. Zuckerman, M. and Lubin, B., *Manual for the Multiple Affect Adjective Check List* (Educational and Industrial Testing Service, San Diego, 1965).

30. Zuckerman, M., 'The Development of an Affect Adjective Check List for the Measurement of Anxiety', *Journal of Consulting Psychology*, **24** (1960), pp. 457–60.

31. Jesness, C. F., *The Jesness Inventory* (Consulting Psychologists Press, Palo Alto, 1966).

32. Vallance, R. C. and Forrest, A. R., 'A Study of the Jesness Personality Inventory with Scottish Children', *British Journal of Educational Psychology*, **41** (1971), pp. 338–44.

33. Bene, E. and Anthony, A. J., *The Family Relations Test* (National Foundation for Educational Research, London, 1957).

34. Goyette, C. H., Conners, C. K. and Ulrich, R. F., 'Normative Data on Revised Conners Parent and Teacher Rating Scales', *Journal of Abnormal Child Psychology*, **6** (1978), pp. 221–36.

35. Stott, D. H., *Bristol Social Adjustment Guides Manual (Fifth Edition): The Social Adjustment of Children* (Hodder and Stoughton, London, 1974).

36. Spivack, G. and Spotts, J. 'The Devereux Child Behavior Scale: Symptom Behaviors in Latency Age Children', *American Journal of Mental Deficiency*, **69** (1965), pp. 839–53.

37. Spivack, G. and Spotts, J., 'Adolescent Symptomatology', *American Journal of Mental Deficiency*, **72** (1967), pp. 74–95.

38. Spivack, G. and Swift, M. S., 'The Devereux Elementary School Behavior Rating Scales: a Study of the Nature and Organisation of Achievement Related Disturbed Classroom Behavior', *Journal of Special Education*, **1** (1966), pp. 71–90.

39. Wirt, R. D., Lacher, D., Klinedinst, J. K. and Seat, P. D., *Multidimensional Description of Child Personality: A Manual for the Personality Inventory for Children* (Western Psychological Services, Los Angeles, 1977).

40. Miller, L. C., Barrett, C. L., Hampe, E. and Noble, H., 'Revised Anxiety Scales for the Louisville Behavior Check List', *Psychological Reports*, **29** (1971), pp. 503–11.

41. Stevenson, H. W. and Odon, R. D., 'The Relation of Anxiety to Children's Performance on Learning and Problem-solving', *Child Development*, **36** (1965), pp. 1003–12.

42. Martin, B., 'The Measurement of Anxiety', *Journal of General Psychology*, **61** (1959), pp. 189–203.

43. Kaufman, A. S., 'Factor Analysis of the WISC-R at Eleven Age Levels Between $6\frac{1}{2}$ and $16\frac{1}{2}$ Years', *Journal of Consulting and Clinical Psychology*, **44** (1975), pp. 135–47.

44. Kaufman, A. S., 'Issues in Psychological Assessment: Interpreting the WISC-R Intelligently' in B. B. Lahey and A. E. Kazdin (eds) *Advances in Clinical*

*Child Psychology*, 3 (Plenum Press, New York, 1977), pp. 177–214.

45. Lutey, C., *Individual Intelligence Testing: A Manual and Source Book* (2nd edn), (Lutey, Colorado, 1977).

46. Wechsler, D., *The Measurement and Appraisal of Adult Intelligence* (Williams and Wilkins, Baltimore, 1958).

47. Venables, P. H., 'Autonomic Reactivity' in M. Rutter (ed.) *Scientific Foundations of Developmental Psychiatry* (Heinemann Medical, London, 1980), pp. 165–75.

48. Venables, P. H., 'Psychophysiology and Psychometrics', *Psychophysiology*, 15 (1978), pp. 302–15.

49. Davies, J. G. V. and Maliphant, R., 'Autonomic Responses of Male Adolescents Exhibiting Refractory Behaviour in School', *Journal of Child Psychology and Psychiatry*, 12 (1971), pp. 115–27.

50. Wade, B. E., 'Highly Anxious Pupils in Formal and Informal Primary Classrooms; the Relationship Between Inferred Coping Strategies and: I Cognitive Attainment: II Classroom Behaviour', *British Journal of Educational Psychology*, 51 (1981), pp. 39–49, 50–7.

51. Cattell, R. B., 'The Nature and Genesis of Mood States' in C. D. Spielberger (ed.) *Anxiety: Current Trends in Theory and Research* (Academic Press, New York, 1972), pp. 115–83.

# 3 RECOGNITION AND TREATMENT OF ANXIETY IN CHILDREN BY MEANS OF PSYCHIATRIC INTERVIEW

Philip Barker

The psychiatric interview is probably the most used and simplest clinical method of assessing anxiety in children. Interviews with children should however always be combined with interviews with the parents or whoever the current care-takers are. The younger the child the more important the parental interview is but it should not be omitted at any age. When dealing with school-aged children it is often advisable to interview also the child's teacher, and at any age there may be other adults with knowledge of the child who can provide useful information.

The psychiatric interview of the child will be dealt with first, following which parental interviews will be discussed. The assessment of anxiety in a child is usually carried out as part of a comprehensive assessment of the child's mental state which, in turn, is normally but part of a wider assessment of the family system, as will be discussed in Chapter 6. There will therefore be many other questions in the interviewer's mind other than whether the child is anxious and about what.

## Interviewing Children

Many accounts of how to conduct psychiatric interviews with children are available, for example those of Stone and Kupernik,[1] Chess and Hassibi,[2] Simmons[3] and Barker.[4] In addition a valuable contribution was made by Rutter and Graham[5] when they carried out a series of studies to investigate the reliability and validity of the psychiatric assessment of children. Their findings will be referred to later.

It will be convenient to describe the interview process under four headings, but these do not represent four separate stages, and all four may be occurring simultaneously.

1. Establishing rapport with the child.
2. Observing the child's behaviour.
3. Talking with the child and learning of the child's thoughts, feelings and ideas.
4. Engaging the child in play.

*Establishing Rapport*

To be in rapport with a person implies the existence of a sympathetic relationship and a state of understanding, harmony and accord. The understanding of course will initially be partial, but in a state of rapport the subject feels that the interviewer has a genuine desire to understand him/her. Verbal and non-verbal means may be used to establish rapport and the skilled interviewer will use both.

*Non-verbal communication* may be more important than verbal in establishing rapport. The way in which the room in which the child is being seen is furnished and arranged is important. Younger children are best seen in a playroom, containing toys and play materials appropriate to the child's age. Indeed all aspects of the interview have to be geared to the child's age and an interviewer's approach to a three-year-old will be very different to that used with a 13-year-old.

The room should thus be child-oriented and there should be a table and chairs appropriate to the child's size available. It is usually helpful not to have a desk, or other items of furniture, between examiner and child. It may be best to face the child directly, but some children feel less threatened when the examiner sits beside them, perhaps at a table, doll's house or sand tray, while making eye contact from time to time. The astute examiner can usually quickly sense which approach is best from the child's initial reaction. The interviewer's mode of dress may be important. If the interviewer is dressed in an immaculate three-piece business suit and tie it may be harder to establish rapport, especially with older children and many teenagers who are rebelling against conventional adult standards. The teenager who comes into the room carrying a package of cigarettes is probably conveying the message that he/she would like to smoke and it may enhance the establishment of rapport if such a wish is allowed — even though the interviewer may deplore the fact that many young people smoke.

Many aspects of the interviewer's behaviour can also be used to help establish rapport. It can be useful to match the child's body posture, rate of breathing, speed of talking, tone of voice, movements and vocabulary. These are all techniques used by hypnotherapists in establishing rapport, but they are equally valuable in routine clinical interviews. The developers of 'Neuro-Linguistic Programming'[6,7] have also pointed out that matching predicates with those of the subject being interviewed can assist. Predicates are words which describe the way things are and include verbs, adjectives, and adverbs. Thus if the subject tends to describe things using visual predicates ('I see what you mean', 'things look bright to me', 'it's like looking at things through a smoke haze', and so on), it is helpful if the interviewer responds with similar visually oriented statements. If the subject uses the auditory mode ('things sound bad to me', 'I hear what you are saying' and so on), then the interviewer should respond with auditory-based statements. Again if the subject uses mainly feeling-type statements ('I feel really burdened down', 'that is a great weight off my shoulders', 'I have a lot of heavy responsibilities', and so on), the interviewer should try and use similar statements in response.

*The content of verbal communication* is also important in establishing rapport. It is important to accept what a child says. Thus a child may voice all kinds of unjustified fears, worries, obsessional thoughts, depressive ideas, values and beliefs which the interviewer may feel tempted to deny. During the stage of establishing rapport, however, it is best to accept the child's view of things. Milton Erickson, perhaps one of the most effective interviewers psychiatry has known, was especially skilled in establishing rapport with his patients and frequently opened his statements by repeating back what the patient had said about his/her feelings or point of view, though often with something additional tagged on. Erickson's way of entering into his patients' worlds is well described by Lankton and Lankton.[8] Certainly the interviewer should not reject any statements presented by the child being interviewed, nor react to them with shock, disagreement or disbelief. Changing the subject's view of the world is a later step in the process of assessment and treatment.

*The use of the child's own language* helps establish rapport and effective communication. The interviewer should find out what terms the child uses, for example, for the male and female sex organs and for masturbation and sexual intercourse. Some key terms may be obtained from the child or adolescent, others may be tried out to discover whether they are understood.

It is sometimes useful to ask for children's help, for example with spelling their names or the names of their schools: this can raise a child's status and self-image in the interview situation.

When subjects are avoided by children being interviewed, or when they have trouble talking freely on a subject, the situation requires careful examination. The topic may be of particular significance to the child. The form of the avoidance, the context in which it occurs and the examiner's own feelings on the subject all bear consideration. If a child has trouble talking about sex, is it because the examiner is ill at ease? Subjects on which an interviewer regularly has trouble getting children to talk may have some special significance to the interviewer.

### Observing the Child's Behaviour

There are many behavioural manifestations of anxiety and it is important to observe the child's physical appearance and behaviour closely throughout the interview. The physical manifestations of anxiety include motor tension, which may be shown by shakiness, trembling, jumpiness, muscle tension, aching muscles, fatiguability, inability to relax, fidgeting, restlessness, and being easily startled; autonomic hyperactivity, which may be shown by sweating, pounding or racing heart, cold, clammy hands, dry mouth, feelings of dizziness or lightheadedness, tingling in hands or feet, the feeling of having an upset stomach, hot or cold spells, frequent urination, diarrhoea, the feeling of having a lump in the throat, flushing, pallor, and raised pulse and respiration rates; and also hypoattentiveness and distractibility, difficulty concentrating, and impatience.

The anxious child is often restless, and may get up and walk around the room inappropriately during the interview. He/she may also find it hard to sustain a conversation on one particular topic or continue with the same line of play or with completion of a drawing or painting.

It is important to take note also of the subjects under discussion, or the material being dealt with in play, drawing or painting, when these behaviours become more, or less marked.

*Separation anxiety* may also be observed. This is manifested by a reluctance to part from, usually, the mother but it may be the father or some other person. An increase in the child's level of anxiety and tension, and perhaps tearfulness, may be evident when attempts are made to have him/her leave the parent or parents in order to be interviewed alone. The management of separation anxiety can be difficult. It can be hard to distinguish between it and a desire on the part of the child to control the interview situation. While both these features may be present, in separation anxiety overt signs of anxiety, as mentioned above, are likely to be more marked than if the child is primarily striving to take control of the interview process. In the latter case anger, or a sullen refusal to cooperate, may be more pronounced.

In managing the reluctance or refusal to separate, various options are available. Adequate preparation of the child helps. It is very desirable that the assessment procedure be explained in advance. This can sometimes be done by the person referring the child, at least if that person is aware of the procedure the psychiatrist follows. Other possibilities are to have the receptionist, secretary or appointments clerk explain to the family what happens and how the child should be prepared; or to send a written explanation in advance of the appointment. It does no harm to do more than one of these things, as long as the explanations given are all the same.

What should the family be told in advance? The most important point is that the assessment is to find out what is troubling the child and the family in order to help put these things right. The main thing to avoid is the idea that the child will be subject to criticism or will in some way be found wanting. This is a real danger since may children are told prior to being brought for assessment, that their behaviour is in one way or another unacceptable, naughty, upsetting to others or in some way 'bad'. As far as possible such messages should not be conveyed to a child who is to be brought for assessment.

*Panic attacks* are another manifestation of anxiety and may be observed when a child is faced with the threat of separation from a parent or other familiar adult. Panic attacks are an acute form of anxiety. They may be caused by some real life-threatening situation, as when a person comes under attack by gunfire or is involved in an earthquake. In such circumstances panic may be an understandable, even normal reaction. Anxious children panic in other, more normal, circumstances. The symptoms characteristic of panic attacks, as set out in the American Psychiatric Association's Diagnostic and Statistical Manual, third edition (DSM-III),[9] are dyspnoea; palpitations; chest pain or discomfort; choking or smothering sensations; dizziness, vertigo, or unsteady feelings;

feelings of unreality; paraesthesia (such as tingling in hands or feet); hot and cold flushes; sweating; faintness; trembling or shaking; and fear of dying, going crazy or doing something uncontrolled.

## Talking with the Child

Much information about the child's level of anxiety can be obtained during conversation. A scheme for interviewing children has been set out elsewhere,[4] but issues which should be covered in conversation with children include their family situation, their school situation, their friends and peer group relationships, their interests, hobbies and sports activities, their concerns, worries, fears and dislikes, any physical symptoms from which they may suffer (anxiety can often be expressed through somatic symptoms), their sleep and any dreams they may experience, and their fantasy life. Once rapport has been established with the child it is often possible to get a conversation going covering various topics and the examiner can look for the manifestations of anxiety mentioned above. They may appear or become more marked when certain topics are spoken about.

The child may report subjective feelings of anxiety, for example, the feeling that the heart is pounding or racing, dizziness, feeling discomfort in the pit of the stomach or a lump in the throat, as well as various worries, fears, or the anticipation of more misfortune befalling self or others. There may be rumination on particular topics and feelings of being 'on edge' and irritable.

Sometimes subjects which are associated with anxiety are specifically avoided during conversation.

Enquiry into a child's fantasy life may prove revealing, where little of substance emerges during other types of conversation. Children may be asked to give three wishes, saying what they would like to happen if, by magic, whatever they wished would come true. They may then come up with things like 'I wish my parents wouldn't separate', having perhaps previously said nothing about this subject; or they may 'wish we had more money', alerting the interviewer to the possibility that the family may have financial problems, or the child may think they have. Similarly children may be asked about the best thing, and the worst thing, in the world that could happen to them; and about who they would like to have with them if they were shipwrecked on a desert island, and why.

The various subjects mentioned above should be raised in a

natural, conversational way in whatever order seems most appropriate for the particular child. It is usually best not to start with the problem area, but to talk first about other aspects of the child's life, working round to the problem areas later. It must be remembered that it is seldom the child who is complaining of symptoms but usually an adult, most often parent or teacher, who is either complaining on the child's behalf or perhaps is objecting to some feature of the child's behaviour. The conversation may start with such relatively neutral topics as how the family got to the clinic or wherever they are being seen, the child's interests and hobbies, any recent birthday or other event, such as Christmas, Easter, Thanksgiving, or a holiday. Gradually the conversation can be steered to other, more emotionally charged, subjects.

The interview should not if possible consist of a series of direct questions; such an approach seldom gives the desired result. It is more a matter of saying 'lots of people have dreams when they are asleep . . . I wonder if you do?' The child who admits to having dreams can then be invited to recount one, and then perhaps be asked whether they are mostly nice or mostly nasty dreams. A child who denies having or remembering dreams may be told 'often when people who don't have dreams come to see us, they like to make up a dream . . . to pretend they have had one . . . perhaps you would like to do that?' Later the interviewer might say something like 'now I would like you to pretend that you are all alone on a desert island (or in a boat) and you could choose one person to be with you . . . anyone you would like but just one person . . . I wonder who you would have?' It is often possible then to get the child to choose a second, then a third person.

Fears, worries, and other symptoms are enquired about in a similar way. Conversation about family, friends (whom the child can be asked to name and describe) and school can be encouraged in much the same way. Throughout this process the interviewer must respond appropriately to what the child is saying, trying to share the child's sorrow at the loss of a pet or pleasure at being a member of a winning football team. Above all it is important always to convey interest in the child's point of view. This does not necessarily imply approving of what the child does or thinks, but disapproval is to be avoided during the diagnostic process — and indeed in therapy also.

*Play*

All children who have not reached adolescence should be given the opportunity to draw, paint, and/or play with some of the available toys and play materials. Their approach to these activities, how well they concentrate and their motor functioning all give useful diagnostic information which may contribute to the interviewer's understanding of how anxious they are. The content of children's play often gives helpful information also. Children who cannot verbalise their anxieties may play them out. Thus a child fearing that he or someone else may die may not verbalise this fear but may play it out in a sand tray or doll's house with family figures or dolls. Puppets may be used in the same way. Anxieties about school, sibling rivalry, peer group relationships, problems in relationships with other adults and many other issues may similarly be played out, or drawn or painted. Time spent playing with children is thus well spent and it is important that the child be made to feel free to use the materials just as he/she wishes.

Adolescents may or may not wish to paint, draw, or play, but some have artistic talents which they are glad to display. Sometimes adolescents will produce poems they have composed at home or paintings they have done previously.

An important feature of children's play, drawing and painting, and indeed to some extent of their conversation too, is the sequence of events. The sequence of activities and issues coming up in play may provide clues as to how things are associated in the child's mind. Thus if, as a child begins to play with a mother figure in the doll's house, aggressive behaviour is displayed, this may indicate feelings of anger towards the person who the figure represents. Thus every action or emotion displayed during play should be considered in its temporal context as well as being a phenomenon of its own right.

## Anxiety and Depression

Sometimes anxiety is complicated by depression, or at least a considerable degree of sadness, in which case crying spells or prolonged tearfulness may predominate. The distinction between anxiety and depression, which of course may co-exist, can also present difficulty. There is nowadays a tendency to make the judgment of whether a depressive condition — or for that matter an anxiety state — is present on the basis of specific clinical criteria. Criteria for depression have been set out in both the ninth edition of the International Classification of Diseases (ICD-9)[10] and in the third edition of the Diagnostic and Statistical Manual of the American Psychiatric Association (DSM-III).[9] The latter has more detailed criteria, with specific operational definitions of each state, though precisely how valid these are is unclear. It is also becoming a more widely established practice to use the same criteria for the diagnosis of depression in children as are used in adults.

DSM-III offers two main categories of depressive disorder which are useful for children. These are 'Major Depressive Episode' and 'Dysthymic Disorder' (or 'Depressive Neurosis').

Consideration of the DSM-III criteria for these conditions can be useful in distinguishing between them and anxiety states. Briefly, the criteria for a major depressive episode are a prominent and relatively persistent mood disturbance characterised by such symptoms as sadness, hopelessness, and feeling low, blue, down in the dumps or irritable. In children under six the mood disturbance may have to be inferred from a persistently sad facial expression. There must also be four of a list of symptoms which include appetite or weight change; sleep disturbance; psychomotor agitation or retardation, or 'hypoactivity' in children under six; loss of interest or pleasure in usual activities, or in children under six signs of apathy; loss of energy or fatigue; feelings of worthlessness, self-reproach or excessive guilt; slow thinking or indecisiveness; and recurrent thoughts of death, suicide, the wish to be dead or suicide attempts.

The principal criteria for dysthymic disorder are that for much of the past year the individual has been bothered by symptoms characteristic of a depressive syndrome, but not of sufficient severity and duration to meet the criteria for a major depressive episode. The manifestations may be intermittent with episodes of depressed mood or marked loss of interest or pleasure in usual activities. There must also be three of a list of symptoms including sleep disturbance; lack of energy or tiredness; feelings of inadequacy; low self-esteem or self-deprecation; decreased effectiveness or productivity at school; decreased attention, concentration, or ability to think clearly; social withdrawal; loss of interest in normally enjoyable activities; irritability or excessive anger, in children often expressed towards parents or care-takers; inability to respond to praise or to rewards; lowered activity level or feeling 'low down';

a pessimistic attitude towards the future or feeling sorry for self; tearfulness or crying; and recurrent thoughts of death or suicide.

DSM-III also has criteria for various anxiety states, including 'panic disorder', 'generalized anxiety disorder', 'obsessive-compulsive disorder', and 'post-traumatic stress disorder'. While space does not permit listing of the detailed criteria as set out in DSM-III, they conform essentially to the description of the various types of anxious children set out in this chapter. Use of the specific criteria set down in DSM-III, and also of the rather less-precise descriptions to be found in ICD-9, can however be useful in clarifying the diagnosis in doubtful cases.

## Parent Interviews

Assessment and treatment usually go better if both parents are involved in the process from the beginning. It is usually best to invite the parents to start by describing the problems which have brought them to the interview or, perhaps better, the changes they are seeking. When they have explained these, any necessary further details should be sought. It is important to establish the severity of the symptoms, the situations in which they occur, or are more or less marked, and the history of their development. It is helpful to get a picture of the 'desired state', that is the situation the parents would like to exist if treatment had been completely successful.

When the parents have covered all their concerns, the interviewer should ask questions about aspects of the child's functioning which have not been mentioned. Questioning should cover the various physical systems of the body, the child's speech and the kinds of things he/she talks about, behaviour in different situations, mood and any mood variations, sleep, attitude towards family, friends, and school, and fantasy life and play. The interviewer will be interested in whether the various features of anxiety mentioned above are present, as well as other aspects of the child's functioning and behaviour. In assessing anxiety important points are the child's mood state, how it varies and under what circumstances, what makes the child happy or sad, how long moods last, and what precipitates mood changes of various types. Parent interviews are described more fully in *Basic Child Psychiatry*.[4] Family assessment, in which the whole family is seen together, is discussed in Chapter 6.

## Special Manifestations of Anxiety

Since anxiety may be expressed indirectly, through the operation of mental defence mechanisms, it is important to enquire for the presence of obsessive-compulsive symptoms, phobias, separation anxiety, hysterical conversion symptoms, and dissociative symptoms.

*Obsessions* are intrusive thoughts and ideas of which the individual cannot be rid despite conscious awareness of their unreasonableness and resistance to them. *Compulsions* are actions resulting from such thoughts: they are repetitive, ritualistic activities which may seem purposeful — for example hand washing — but they are carried out needlessly, because of a 'magical' belief that they will prevent some undesirable thing from happening or otherwise influence the course of events. These symptoms are unwelcome, unpleasant and disturbing to the individual. Obsessional thoughts may be shared with the parents by the child and compulsive actions are usually readily observed.

*Phobias* are specific, severe fears of particular objects or situations, for example, animals, heights, open spaces, crowds, crossing bridges and so on. Phobias may be monosymptomatic or there may be a variety of phobic objects.

*Separation anxiety* is manifest when a child is separated from some person with whom he/she has close emotional bonds, or when attempts are made to separate the child. It is often prominent in neurotic school refusal, in which the child develops an irrational fear of leaving home to go to school. DSM-III has a special diagnostic category entitled 'Separation Anxiety Disorder'.

*Hysterical conversion symptoms* consist of the loss or alteration of physical functioning as a result of anxiety which is repressed and then expressed indirectly in this way. The physical manifestations may result from the 'conversion' of anxiety into the symptom or they may be a means of avoiding anxiety-provoking situations. The symptoms may be motor (paralysis or weakness or inability to speak except in a whisper) or sensory (lack of sensation to pain or touch in some part of the body, or the presence of pain, discomfort, or other sensations). Hysterical seizures, blackouts and loss of memory may also occur.

*Dissociative states* include psychogenic fugue, in which the subject wanders away from home or work for a period and engages in apparently purposeful activities, with inability to remember the past; depersonalisation disorder, in which the subject has a feeling of unreality about the self or the environment; and multiple personality. All these are rare in childhood. DSM-III also classifies psychogenic memory loss as a Dissociative Disorder.

Careful enquiry should be made about the child's sleep, since anxious children often suffer from sleep disturbance, particularly insomnia. There may be difficulty in getting to sleep, and/or the child may wake at intervals during the night. It is important to enquire whether the pattern of sleep has changed as other symptoms of anxiety have appeared, or whether the sleep pattern is a longstanding one. The insomnia may be more marked at certain times. Thus the child anxious about going to school may sleep well during school holidays, or sleep disturbance may be more severe when the parents have had a row, in families where marital discord is a factor causing anxiety, or following drinking bouts where there are alcoholic members in the family.

Two special forms of sleep disturbance are *nightmares* and *night terrors*. In night terrors the child wakes up in a frightened, even terrified condition and is inaccessible and does not respond when spoken to. The subject may appear unaware of his/her surroundings and may seem auditorily or visually hallucinated, talking to and looking at people and things not actually there. A characteristic of night terrors is that the child has no recollection of them in the morning; they usually subside in 10 to 15 minutes, during which they may cause great alarm to parents. Night terrors are a normal phenomenon, particularly in children of pre-school age, but it does seem that they may become more frequent and severe in anxious children.

Nightmares are unpleasant dreams which may or may not lead to the child waking up. The striking picture of a disorientated, hallucinated child seen in night terrors is not present, and the child normally has some recollection of the dream in the morning. Nightmares also occur in normal children, but may be more frequent, and their content may be of particular significance, in anxious children.

## Evaluation of Interview Data

When a child and parents, and preferably also the whole family group (see Chapter 6), have been interviewed, the data obtained must be integrated and evaluated. The maifestations of anxiety differ according to the child's age. Pre-school children seldom state that they are anxious, so the presence of anxiety must be inferred from their behaviour. Specific fears are extremely common in children aged four or five. They are accociated with the process of learning about the world and the various things in it. Thus there may be an inordinate fear of insects, dogs, thunder and many other things during this time, though these are usually transitory as the child begins to discover what is dangerous and what is not. Pathological anxiety may be manifest by an excess of such fears, but often has to be inferred as a result of sleep disturbance, restlessness, clinging to parents and other non-verbal behaviour which has been mentioned above. Also important is the developmental sequence of symptoms. In what situation was the anxiety first manifested? How did the symptoms develop and in what situations? How did people react to the child's anxiety — since an over-anxious reaction can reinforce anxiety still further?

Older children are more likely to express their worries verbally, as well as showing the non-verbal manifestations which have been mentioned. Sometimes their anxiety is, at least in part, repressed and expressed through the operation of mental defence mechanisms, as when children present with obsessive-compulsive conditions, hysterical and dissociative phenomena and phobic behaviour. In middle childhood, however, these defence processes are often not well developed and it usually proves relatively easy to penetrate them and discover something about the true nature of the child's worries. In adolescence this is less often the case and defences may be more firmly established. On the other hand, adolescents are often able to discuss their situation, and their fears and worries, in a more adult and graphic way.

The manifestations of anxiety in children should always be considered along with the child's social situation, which includes the situation at school. Under some circumstances anxiety is appropriate. If there is a seriously ill parent, danger the parents may separate, financial instability, difficulty in coping with school work because of a learning problem or other similar stress, a measure of anxiety is to be expected. The interviewer must always be able to form a judgment as to whether the degree of anxiety shown is commensurate with the stress being faced by the child.

## The Reliability and Validity of Interview Techniques

There have been few scientific studies of how reliable and valid is the assessment of children's anxiety by psychiatric interview. Rutter and Graham,[5] however, reported four studies, two of them on children seen in the Isle of Wight epidemiological survey and two on children seen at the Maudsley Hospital, London. The main conclusions were that a standardised half-hour interview with a child can determine whether or not a psychiatric disorder is present with a reasonable degree of reliability. The interview proved to be less satisfactory when particular features of psychiatric disorders were considered, though the rating of anxiety was found to be more reliable than that of depression. It appears from this study that some of the commonly accepted indicators of anxiety, for example, fidgetiness, tension, and tremulousness (which proved an uncommon phenomenon in children aged nine to twelve) are of marginal value. An anxious expression, a pre-occupation with anxiety topics and apprehension on entering the interview room, on the other hand, were significantly more frequent in neurotic children than among the control group.

There have been more extensive studies of parent interviews. Graham and Rutter[11] describe a study in which parents of 268 children were interviewed using a standard interview schedule. This was also part of the Isle of Wight epidemiological study of ten- and twelve-year-olds. Again the interview appeared to provide a reliable assessment of behaviour during the previous year, and also of the presence or absence of psychiatric abnormality, but the specific issue of judging the degree of anxiety present in a child was not addressed in this study. A later series of six papers by Rutter and his colleagues[12-17] reported on studies of parent interviews done at the Maudsley Hospital. While none of these addressed specifically the eliciting of symptoms of anxiety in the children, they did provide much useful information about how to elicit feelings and facts in parent interviews. The data on how to elicit facts are more relevant to the assessment of anxiety symptoms in children than those dealing with mothers' feelings. When encouraged to talk freely, most mothers seeking help with their children's problems mentioned most, but not all, of the key issues. Some were not mentioned and the quality and detail of the information provided were often imperfect. More systematic questioning can yield rather more information. If less active and less structured styles are used, specific detailed questioning and probing are essential. Open-ended questions such as 'how did your son show that he felt miserable?' or 'tell me more about how he was feeling' are more effective than closed ones such as 'did he cry?' or 'how many times did he say he felt he couldn't go on any longer?' It can also be helpful to check back that the interviewer has properly understood the reply, at the same time inviting clarification. Use of the information provided in these papers should increase the efficiency with which symptoms of anxiety in children are elicited from parents.

## Treatment of Anxiety in Children by Psychiatric Interview

This section will deal only with calming techniques which may be used in the course of a psychiatric interview. The possible causes of anxiety are many and they may be complex, as will be clear from the other chapters in this book. The psychiatric interview itself, as opposed to the various forms of psychotherapy, and other treatments, is not usually the mainstay of a treatment plan. Nevertheless it is helpful if the interviewer can take appropriate steps to deal with anxiety which is detected during the interview. Sometimes milder forms of anxiety, including some of those which are reactions to recent events, can be helped and certainly it should be possible for the interviewer to assist the child in dealing with anxiety related to the interview situation itself.

There are three groups of simple techniques which may be useful in calming anxious children at interview.

1. Empathic listening and acceptance of what the child has to tell about his/her worries.
2. Exploration of the child's situation, and the cause of any anxiety he/she may be experiencing, with discussion of how the circumstances have made the child anxious and what simple methods the child might take to deal with the situation.
3. Specific anxiety-relieving techniques such as 'reframing' and certain other techniques developed by the originators of Neuro-Linguistic Programming (NLP).

### Empathic Listening

We are all familiar with the way we often feel better after we have spoken to an accepting, understanding, and empathic person about something that is worrying us. An old adage says 'a trouble shared is a trouble halved', and this applies as much to talking to children about their worries and fears as it does to any other situation. For some children it is a new experience to be listened to and given the full attention of an accepting adult; once children find that what they say is accepted and the therapist is not overwhelmed or shocked, this may reduce the intensity of their anxiety. It may be helpful to respond with statements like, 'Wow, that must have been scary' or 'I wonder how that made you feel, you can't have been expecting that sort of thing to happen?'

Discussion of the child's worries, and the context in which they have arisen, may itself help, by providing the child with a new perspective on the situation. This probably accounts for the considerable improvement which sometimes follows a single interview, even one intended primarily as diagnostic. Anxiety arising from the interview itself can often be alleviated by an explanation of the purpose of the interview and of how the interviewer aims to help deal with whatever is troubling the child.

## Exploring the Child's Situation

Simply discussing the situation in an empathic way is often, of course, insufficient to relieve the child's anxiety. In such cases some further exploration and discussion of the implications of the things which are worrying the child and discussion also of possible ways of handling the situation may be useful. Anxiety can build on itself and the tense child, feeling under pressure, may find it hard to view things objectively. Sometimes anxiety arises from the misinterpretation of things the child has heard. Thus a girl on one occasion heard her parents arguing in their bedroom about whether or not they should get rid of 'her'. She immediately assumed that they were discussing her, since she had earlier been reprimanded for some minor misdeeds, and became acutely anxious lest she was to be cast out of the family. It transpired however that the parents were discussing whether or not to get rid of their dog — actually it was a bitch! Children sometimes misinterpret things such as the severity and implications of family members' illnesses, their parents' work difficulties, issues concerning the family pets and a multitude of other things.

Often, of course, there is a real cause for anxiety. In such cases it may be helpful to discuss with the child alternatives available to both the child and other family members, in dealing with their situation. Realising that there are a number of constructive and viable alternatives available may again help relieve the child's anxiety considerably. It can be helpful to tell the child stories about other children who have been in similar situations and who, either by their own efforts or by the efforts of the family or others, survived a period of anxiety and emerged stronger as a result. Self-disclosure can be useful here. While psychiatrists differ as to how far self disclosure is appropriate in psychiatric interviews, it should not be ruled out as a potentially helpful device. It may well be that the interviewer has had an experience similar to the child's and went through a period of anxiety which was in some way or other resolved. It may be useful to share this with the child. Or the interviewer may be able to share with the child an experience of one of his/her own children or other family members, describing how this was dealt with and leading to a happy outcome.

## Neuro-Linguistic Programming

'Reframing' can be a very useful technique. It is discussed helpfully in a book of that name by Grinder and Bandler.[18] Many circumstances and behaviours can be reframed, so that they come to have a new meaning. Shannon, an eleven-year-old-girl, was prone to tell frequent lies. At interview she was found to be tense and anxious, apparently because of much disapproval from parents and teacher. She had been subject to increasing criticism and punishment, so that she was feeling very much the odd person out in the family and presented the picture of a very worried child, with a little superimposed depression. Once the situation became clear to the interviewer, he spent some time reframing lying as a very valuable asset. 'I really admire the way you are able to think up new, and exciting things to tell people. I wish I had such a rich imagination', he told Shannon. The many advantages of being able to make up new, creative and convincing stories were discussed. Such, after all, is what makes great short story writers and novelists. By the end of the session the child's capacity to make up stories had been reframed as valuable, the question then becoming that of determining the situations in which this asset would be useful, as opposed to those in which it would not. A similar line was taken in subsequent family interviews and the upshot was both a decrease in the child's anxiety and the virtual disappearance of the pathological lying. Instead the child was encouraged by the therapist to write short stories from imagination and these were highly praised as they were indeed excellent compositions.

The developers of Neuro-Linguistic Programming (NPL)[6,7] techniques have described a number of relatively simple techniques which can produce changes in individuals quickly and economically. While reframing is one of these, its essence is to give a different meaning, often a more hopeful or acceptable one, to something which might previously have been a source of anxiety or concern.

Other NLP procedures involve the use of 'anchoring'. This term is used for the phenomenon whereby specific sensory experiences become associated with particular events, behaviours and ways of reacting to situations. People have known, probably from time immemorial, that paricular sensory stimuli can evoke whole memories and can cause a person to recall complex past events. Thus a piece of music can bring back to us a vivid memory of some past experience and our reaction to it. Yet the music was only a tiny part of that experience. It was however one which became an anchor for the experience. In *Frogs into Princes*[7] Bandler and Grinder describe how, after rapport has been established with a subject, a particular state of behaviour and feeling may be anchored by having the person re-experience, in fantasy, the visual, auditory and feeling sensations which were present. This state is then anchored by, for example, touching the person on the wrist or elbow or elsewhere. First such an anchor is firmly established, for example for an experience to which the subject reacts in an anxious way, so that the state is promptly recalled when the anchor is fired. Then another past experience, perhaps of an incompatible state, for example one in which the subject experienced confidence, joy, and happiness, is anchored in the same way, though of course the tactile anchor will be in a different situation. It has been found that if the two anchors are then 'collapsed', that is to say fired at the same time, the subject will have more choice in responding in similar situations to the one which originally stimulated anxiety. In other words the subject will have available to him/her the possibility of being confident and joyful, rather than anxious. The effectiveness of the procedure can immediately be tested by 'future pacing' the subject. This involves having the subject fantasise, using the three principal sensory modalities, a future event which in the past provoked anxiety. Then, preferably while firing the anchor for confident feelings, the person can discover whether or not it is now possible to deal with this situation in a different way.

A number of other NLP techniques, some of them rather more complex, are available to deal with anxiety. One, known as 'changed personal history', consists of having the subject re-experience, in fantasy, a series of past unsatisfactory — perhaps anxiety-provoking — experiences. These are re-experienced in turn, working backwards from the most recent to the very first occasion. Each time the subject re-lives the visual, auditory and feeling experiences of the event. Next the resources required to deal with these situations in a different, and more adaptive, way are then identified. These will often be occasions in the subject's life when a confident, mature, and certainly non-anxious state was experienced. The subject is then asked to re-experience, again in fantasy, an occasion on which these resources were used. If no such occasion can be identified, the subject can be asked to model some-one else who has displayed the behaviours required. The events previously relived in fantasy are then gone over again, but this time with the addition of the new resource. Thus the subject goes into, and experiences in fantasy (or what is really a hypnotic trance), the previous events but with the crucial difference that there is the additional resource now available. Sometimes several different resources have to be identified, if the subject cannot handle the situations with the aid of a single resource. In that case the anchor is 'stacked' until the subject can experience the events, in fantasy, in a completely satisfactory and non-anxious way.

Other NLP techniques are available to deal with phobias and the effect of past discrete traumatic experiences. All are applicable to children although their use with younger children requires creative use of the basic principles of and the capacity to communicate effectively with children of the ages concerned.

**Summary and Conclusions**

Anxiety is a universal experience in children, but sometimes it becomes excessive and threatens to, or actually does, overwhelm the child so that adaptive functioning is compromised. The clinical psychiatric interview is a useful and commonly employed method of assessing whether anxiety is present in children, and if so what are its severity and causes. The interview should start with the establishment of rapport, and information can then be obtained from the behaviour, content of talk and play of the child. This information should always be complemented by a detailed history of the child's symptoms and reactions from the parents and other adults with an intimate knowledge of him. An interview with the whole family is also helpful. Discussion of the child's worries, and the issues behind them, in a supportive and empathic way, with explanation of how the problems have arisen and may be alleviated, can help reduce or even remove excessive anxiety. In addition there are a number of specific techniques which can allow children to obtain access to the resources they require to deal with situations more effectively. Several of these can be incorporated within a psychiatric interview. In some cases anxiety in children is a symptom of a more serious disorder. These cases require more specialised treatment, usually treatment programmes that will attack the underlying disorders.

## References

1. Stone, F. H. and Kupernik, C., *Child Psychiatry for Students* (Churchill Livingstone, Edinburgh, 1974).

2. Chess, S. and Hassibi, M., *Principles and Practice of Child Psychiatry* (Plenum, New York, 1978).

3. Simmons, J. E., *Psychiatric Examination of Children*, 3rd edn (Lea and Febiger, Philadelphia, 1981).

4. Barker, P., *Basic Child Psychiatry*, 4th edn (Granada, St. Albans, 1983).

5. Rutter, M. and Graham, P., 'The Reliability and Validity of the Psychiatric Assessment of the Child: I. Interview with the Child', *British Journal of Psychiatry, 114* (1968), pp. 563–79.

6. Dilts, R., Grinder, J., Bandler, R., Bandler, L. C. and Delozier, J., *Neuro-Linguistic Programming*, vol. 1 (Meta Publications, Cupertino, CA, 1980).

7. Bandler, R. and Grinder, J., *Frogs into Princes* (Real People Press, Moab, Utah, 1979).

8. Lankton, S. R. and Lankton, C. H., *The Answer Within: A Clinical Framework of Ericksonian Hypnotherapy* (Brunner/Mazel, New York, 1983).

9. American Psychiatric Association, *Diagnostic and Statistical Manual III* (APA, Washington, D.C., 1980).

10. World Health Organisation, *International Classification of Diseases, 1975 Revision* (WHO, Geneva, 1977).

11. Graham, P. and Rutter, M., 'The Reliability and Validity of the Psychiatric Assesment of the Child: 2. Interview with the Parent', *British Journal of Psychiatry, 114* (1968), pp. 581–92.

12. Rutter, M. and Cox, A. 'Psychiatric Interviewing Techniques: 1. Methods and Measures', *British Journal of Psychiatry, 138* (1981), pp. 273–82.

13. Cox, A., Hopkinson, K. and Rutter, M., 'Psychiatric Interviewing Techniques II. Naturalistic Study: Eliciting Factual Information', *British Journal of Psychiatry, 138* (1981), pp. 283–91.

14. Hopkinson, K., Cox, A. and Rutter, M., 'Psychiatric Interviewing

Techniques III. Naturalistic Study: Eliciting Feelings', *British Journal of Psychiatry, 138* (1981), pp. 406–15.

15. Rutter, M. and Cox, A. *et al.*, 'Psychiatric Interviewing Techniques IV. Experimental Study: Four Contrasting Styles', *British Journal of Psychiatry, 138* (1983), pp. 456–65.

16. Cox, A., Rutter, M. and Holbrook, D., 'Psychiatric Interviewing Techniques V. Experimental Study: Eliciting Factual Information', *British Journal of Psychiatry, 139* (1981), pp. 29–37.

17. Cox, A., Holbrook, D. and Rutter, M., 'Psychiatric Interviewing Techniques VI. Experimental Study: Eliciting Feelings', *British Journal of Psychiatry, 139* (1981), pp. 144–52.

18. Grinder, J. and Bandler, R., *Reframing: Neuro-Linguistic Programming and the Transformation of Meaning* (Real People Press, Moab, Utah, 1983).

# 4 THE CONTRIBUTION OF PROJECTIVE TECHNIQUES TO THE RECOGNITION AND MONITORING OF ANXIETY IN SCHOOL CHILDREN

Elsie L. Osborne

## Introduction

Much of the early work in the development of projective techniques was carried out in relation to adults, especially in clinical situations, where such techniques made a major contribution to the psychologists' understanding of individual problems of adjustment.

Amongst those who extended their use to work with children, a special contribution was made by Jessie Francis-Williams, formerly consultant psychologist to Guy's Hospital, London, with long experience in residential and non-residential children's settings.

Some of the material for this chapter originates in notes which Jessie Francis-Williams left for possible publication before her death in July 1977. Her studies of the effects of early deprivation and separation, through hospitalisation, neglect or abandonment, and generally of children in care were outstanding and her book on the Rorschach with children[1] remains the primary reference work in this field.

This chapter is, therefore, an acknowledgement of a personal debt to her as teacher and colleague over many years, as well as of this particular contribution.

Many accounts of the theory or rationale of projective psychology are contained in the literature and readers are referred to these for details. They are often linked to a specific technique and the approach varies from one author to another. Examples include Theodora Alcock,[2] Herbert Phillipson[3,4] and Abt and Bellak.[5]

In general rationales are based on a psychodynamic approach with support from theories of perception.[6] What is common to them all is the notion of perception as a selective process in which many factors are involved, including an emotional basis. This dynamic process of organising experience reflects the individual's unique personality. Psychoanalytic theories of projection

56

emphasise the need to take account of unconscious as well as conscious dynamics, especially as they influence relationships.

The techniques themselves provide an opportunity for a sampling of these processes in the expectation that the responses made will be characteristic of other occasions and situations. Whilst such responses are, of course, mediated by intelligence and awareness of external reality (in this case the technique material and the setting in which it is being given), there is an important contribution to the clinician's understanding in that the techniques also give access to material about feelings which could often not be directly communicated.

## Projective Techniques in Use with Children

The techniques most commonly in use with very young children include those where the child is invited to play with some attractive material, for example, the Lowenfeld[7] world play of miniature toys, and the London Doll Play material.[8]

Most techniques in use with school age children require a more verbal kind of response and it is with these that this chapter is mainly concerned. Among these the most popular would certainly include the Children's Apperception Test (the CAT) developed by Bellak and Bellak[9] which has been very much used with children of primary school age. Like many others, including Murray's well known Thematic Apperception Test (TAT)[9] on which it was based, the CAT uses a set of pictures about which the child is invited to tell stories. The TAT is still used with children but with adolescents (from about 13 years onwards) it has to a large extent been replaced by the Object Relations Techniques (ORT).[4]

Perhaps the most famous of all projective techniques is the Rorschach 'ink blot' test, the use of which with children and adolescents has been explored at length. Apart from the book by Jessie Francis-Williams to which reference has already been made,[1] normative studies have been made by Ames *et al.* of 2 to 10 year olds[10] and 10 to 16 year olds,[11] and a more clinical approach elaborated by Halpern.[12]

### Developments in the Use of Projective Techniques

The list above could be extended much further and the reader may check for an overall review of projective techniques with children in Rabin and Haworth.[13] Since then further additions have been made. One of these, the Pickford Projective Pictures,[14] has made more explicit the therapeutic possibilities of a picture/story technique in contrast to the assessment and differential diagnosis emphasised previously. Although often used as a preliminary to recommendation for psychotherapy or other help it was a long time before the potential of such techniques as therapeutic instruments in themselves was fully appreciated. In the case of the Pickford pictures this was achieved by having a much larger selection of pictures available so that they might be used over a fairly long series of sessions.

It was my own experience, however, that an administration of one of the shorter techniques in a single session seemed often to be therapeutic in itself or could provide a basis for discussion in subsequent meetings through highlighting and clarifying major areas of anxiety.

The process of responding to the pictures, blots or other material, in the presence of an accepting adult, was frequently seen to be an experience which was releasing and yet also reassuring. This is illustrated in many cases by a child's hesitant start, requests to have everything confirmed before continuing, tentative suggestions and much checking back with the psychologist or therapist, followed by increasing freedom, originality and enjoyment.

Of course the attitude of the psychologist is an important factor but it is also not unusual for some children to be unable to respond directly even to a very sympathetic counsellor, and to hold back from revealing the very things that worry them most. Helping to meet this situation is a significant contribution of projective techniques in the understanding of children's anxieties. They provide material which allows children to reveal themselves at one remove rather than in a direct confrontation of their fears or distress.

This idea of working indirectly with a child's anxieties is an important one for psychologists who may not be able to undertake long periods of supportive counselling or psychotherapy. They need to find a comparatively rapid way in to an understanding of the underlying feelings, which yet will respect a child's reserves or defences and ensure that the feelings aroused can continue to be contained within the sessions. That is to say, anxieties are not evoked for their own sake, nor allowed to spill out in an uncontrollable way.

It is also important to bear in mind that the clues as to the nature of the anxieties, provided by the particular technique, may be unconscious and therefore not in the child's awareness in that form. For example, confusion over sexual identity or concern about parental rejection. Such possibilities would most certainly not be raised directly in the first instance. The aim is not to discover a child's secret life but to obtain guidance on the strength of the anxieties and the extent to which they interfere with functioning and a reasonable degree of adjustment in work and relationships. Of equal importance is the understanding of strengths such as flexibility and motivation to manage and to overcome difficulties.

The psychologists' use of the material will depend upon clinical judgment of what will be helpful to the child, which may mean holding on to some hypotheses until the moment seems appropriate to explore them further.

**What is Normal?**

The emphasis in the use of projective techniques on the listing of indicators and the making of differential diagnoses has lessened, although it remains useful to know how the problems encountered by some specifically handicapped groups are likely to influence the way they respond, or of how, for instance, the responses to the Rorschach cards typically change over the years in school age children. Such information is the normative data of projective 'testing' and allows the psychologist to be more alert to the idiosyncrasies of a particular record.

The nature of such unique or unusual features of a record can indicate the extent to which a child sees the world in the same terms, or similar ones at least, to his peers. Where he does not do this the question is raised as to whether what he sees can be reasonably related to the 'reality' provided by the picture or blot or is quite removed from it. Even the most creative response should derive, in some way, from the stimulus material if the child is to be able to share his view of the world with others. Where a number of responses are so strange that they cannot be communicated as in any way relating to the material or are really bizarre rather than individualistic, then it is difficult to see how such a child could make appropriate use of a classroom situation. This may throw new light on a child who is isolated or withdrawn in class.

Such extreme examples of inability to function are comparatively rare, but very important to understand. They represent a borderline close to autism, although even here a more complete look at the overall strengths and weaknesses, at the nature and content of the actual anxieties, must modify and supplement the psychologist's opinion, rather than lead to automatic categorisation or decisions about placement outside of normal school.

### Moira: An Example of the Use of the Rorschach

Moira, at 9 years old, was causing her primary school teacher considerable concern. She explained that Moira was functioning at an educationally subnormal (ESN) level but the teacher was not really happy with such a definition as Moira could read quite fluently and occasionally showed other glimpses of a surprisingly good ability. However, she was withdrawn, difficult to make contact with and complained that she was teased by the other children. The teacher observed that she had in fact no friends.

The information obtained from an intelligence test was useful in that it confirmed that Moira's available ability was at least average, but the results were limited by her wary and suspicious attitude and, therefore, resistance to any attempt to discuss her difficulties.

She responded well to the Rorschach, however, seeming interested and stimulated by it, although she still kept the interviewer at a distance, looking away from her and quite often ignoring her comments and questions.

For a full account of the method of scoring and interpreting a Rorschach record it would be necessary to refer to one of the standard texts. The most widely used in the UK is Klopfer.[15] A more recent publication draws on experience with a number of scoring systems.[16] The method requires consideration to be given not only to the content of the responses made to the ink blots but also to various aspects which can be quantified. These may be summarised as answering the following questions: what is seen? (people, animals, landscapes, objects of various kinds); how is it seen? (in movement, using colour or texture, clearly and in detail etc.) and with what justification in relation to the blot? (making imaginative and appropriate use of details) and where? (in what part of the blot).

In Moira's case a look at the nature of her responses included many monsters, and many wild but unspecified animals, some with spikes, others in a rage or with fire coming from eyes, nose and mouth. Somtimes the monsters were fighting, digging in their nails and sometimes they were incomplete or split. In some cases Moira changed her mind, e.g. an animal changed to a puppet or two girls who seemed quite clearly seen (card 7 of the series, where this is often the case), later became monsters. The other striking features were the strange relationships sometimes described. The monster girls of card 7 were standing on top of a butterfly, and this was justified by saying 'they must be light'. These two responses (of the girls, and of the butterfly) are commonly seen but usually quite distinct. Card 8 also illustrates how Moira could respond adequately to the main features of a blot but then embellished it in a way which hovered close to bizarre. To see two animals and a mountain on this card is very common, and they are often elaborated in an original or creative way in specifying the sort of animals and what they are doing. Moira did not specify the kind of animals but said that the mountain was walking and the animals were holding its hand.

The view of Moira's world which emerges is frightening and strange. She responds in a fairly accurate or realistic way to the broad outlines of what is presented to her, but what she adds from her own imagination is almost invariably unreal and often persecutory. There were more positive features, in that she struggled to deal with the task, specifying some things she could not account for, maybe the colour or some aspect of the shading, e.g. 'There's a black line,' 'The monster should have a hand there, but it's wrong,' 'The animals are red' (these are on card 8 which are of a pink colour in fact although she did not specify what animals they could be) and so on. Looking at the overall quantifiable aspects too, produces a result similar to that which might usually be expected from a child of her age, i.e. a fair mixture of use of colour and movement, although here too there are some unusual features, including considerably more reference to the black as colouring, and a disproportionately large number of responses whenever colour was introduced.

The suggestion therefore was that she could use her intelligence to cope with many of her teacher's demands, where these were unambiguous and did not involve relating to other people, that she was very sentitive to any highly charged emotional impact from the environment and therefore much less able to manage in a normal, lively classroom. Her vulnerability to anything at all threatening was noted and subsequent observation confirmed that she was indeed rejected by the other children because of her own provocative behaviour. The Rorschach record would indicate that this was a defensive manoeuvre to offset any possibility of attack.

The work with the Rorschach provided a basis on which some contact with Moira could be maintained. Regular meetings with her teacher confirmed the help she was also obtaining in class. Her remaining 18 months or so in primary school was therefore reasonably contained but the question of transfer to secondary school was a crucial issue.

It was clearly not appropriate to recommend ESN school but the evidence for her managing in a large secondary school was not encouraging. The concern was that her anxiety would become unmanageable and her hold on reality become less certain once she left the greater security of her very supportive primary school.

Nevertheless in response to considerable parental pressures and Moira's own wishes the secondary school felt she should be given a chance to settle there. Indeed in the first term the school reported no problems, it seemed that she could lose herself in its more anonymous atmosphere. This could not be sustained and in the second term there were increasing complaints about her hostility to other children. Eventually the school felt they were unable to contain her much longer. The continued contact with the family meant that an agreement could be reached for transfer to a small special school before the situation had deteriorated to the point of exclusion from school. In the special school Moira subsequently made a good improvement.

**The Use of Projective Techniques in Interviews with a 6 Year Old**

The previous example draws on the diagnostic contribution of the Rorschach to school placement, in particular in assessing the extent of disturbance to normal functioning.

Among the accounts of work with projective techniques which Jessie Francis-Williams left unpublished, is the following example of a little boy called Joseph. It would be unusal to give so many projective techniques to the same child and this example is included, not only for its interest as a procedure for interviewing a very young child, but for the comparisons between the three techniques used.

The first of these, the Bene-Anthony test, suggested the issues involved and the extent to which feelings were denied. Its material is under fairly conscious control by the child. The Rorschach confirmed the Bene-Anthony material but gave more indications of the nature of Joseph's frightening world. Finally the content of his anxieties was opened up in the Rorschach and made even more explicit in the CAT.

Joseph was the oldest child of a London docker. The family lived in a 'high rise' block of flats in the East end of London. Joseph was referred to a clinic because he had been excluded from school for his wild, uncontrollable behaviour and for constant soiling since he absolutely refused to use the toilet. Joseph was rough and in play greatly frightened other children. He lived on the twentieth floor of the flats, but he was not allowed to go down to play with the other children because he was too disruptive. The situation was the same in his infants' school. At play, all the children were afraid of him because he bullied them so roughly. His soiling also made a big problem for his teacher. For these reasons, finally he was excluded from school.

He came to the hospital a clean, tidy, friendly little boy whose overt behaviour made it very hard to see how he could in any way be related to the boy described in the referral letter. His mother said *she* could manage him and that when he was with her he presented no problem. He was a boy of average intelligence and it seemed that there were no basic learning problems. He was given the Bene-Anthony Family Relations Test[17] in order to investigate his relationships and feelings about his family. Joseph happily set up the figures that could represent his own family — father, mother, Joseph himself, Jacqueline his younger sister, and Sam the youngest brother, and the figure which represented 'Nobody'.

In this test the child is given sets of small postcards which are to be posted into the figures selected. The series of postcards carry messages which are designed to express positive feelings coming from the child, negative feelings coming from the child, positive feelings going towards the child, negative feelings going towards the child, and finally feelings of dependence. An analysis of the results of this test showed a very strong denial of feelings of regard by Joseph, a denial also of feelings of dependency. When posting expressions of dependency into 'Nobody', Joseph said, 'Children should learn to look after themselves, shouldn't they?' All the messages expressing dependence, such as, for example, 'Joseph likes you to be with him when he is not feeling well. Who is it Joseph wants when he is not well?' or 'Joseph wants you to come when he is frightened. Who is it Joseph wants when he is frightened?' were posted to 'Nobody'.

To his father he posted many expressions of negative feelings, such as, 'Joseph wants you to go away. Who would Joseph send away?' and to his mother, 'Joseph hates you. Who is it that Joseph hates?' and also, 'You don't like Joseph. Who doesn't like Joseph?'.

Most unusually, Joseph expressed no feeling, positive or negative to either his brother or his sister. The whole presentation showed such a denial of feeling on the part of this boy that it seemed that it would be useful to explore further.

While appearing reasonably co-operative in accepting the Rorschach, his total production was very limited. His main responses were 'legs,' usually bent or twisted; prickly things; worms that have been trodden on and all bleeding, or frightening animals, crocodiles with open mouths ready to bite. His only human response was 'Two people's hands' seen on card 3. His favourite card was 4 which he said was a 'King's Badge'. He liked it but could not elaborate on it at all.

The overall impression was of a child who sees his world as hostile and frightening. To the last card he gave four responses. This is a multicoloured card, more split up than any other. Joseph saw the usual rabbit but with an unusual addition: 'A bunny rabbit's face with long eyes sticking out'. He saw also a spider or daddylonglegs, and a funny old leg bent over. He added, 'I suppose it's a crab'. All of these are common responses. Then he added, 'A pipe with ears'. Subsequently he said that this was the worst card for him. When asked why he disliked it, he said it was horrid and it frightened him. Trying to get an explanation of this really obvious fear and dislike he said, 'It's the pipe . . . with ears'.

He then went on to say, 'It goes down in a lavatory and listens to people. If they've been naughty it makes their ears little and thin and their legs big and fat. It scratches people when it sees them — comes up bang and bites and hits them.' When asked, 'Who told you that?' or 'What makes you think that?', he remained very quiet for a time, obviously quite disturbed by it all and then he said, 'My Mum knows about it. That's why she tries to make me sit on the lavatory. She hates me and would like me to be scratched and hurt.'

This boy's responses to the two projective techniques made it possible for him to present his problems which were giving rise to considerable anxiety and fears of rejection in which much of his behaviour disorder was rooted.

Over a series of sessions he was encouraged to continue to explore these. As he talked most readily through the indirect means of the projective test he was also given the CAT. In this technique, ten pictures developed by Bellak and Bellak[9] were designed to represent situations such as eating, sleeping, fear of loneliness, fantasies about aggression, anxieties regarding parent relation-ships, sibling jealousy.

On the assumption that young children can generally identify more easily and express more freely feelings related to animals than in relation to human beings, these situations are all represented by animals. It is thought that in the child's response to the pictures he would express something of his own ways of reacting to and coping with his own problems of growth in early childhood.

The same theme of rejection ran through the stories Joseph told. The last card represents a toilet scene in which a parent dog is trying to make the puppy use the lavatory. To this Joseph said, 'She's his Mum and she's trying to make him sit on the lavatory but he knows about that pipe with ears and he won't go'. When he was asked what would happen he said, 'His Mum smacked him. Then she took a knife and 'sticked' into his eyes and threw him downstairs without feeling sorry.' This kind of theme ran through all his stories — of parents trying to get rid of their children.

Card 1 shows three little chicks sitting at the table on which is a large bowl of food from which each chick has food in a bowl of his own. From behind is a very shadowy figure of a mother hen. Seeing this Joseph said, 'That's a cuckoo,' pointing to the distant hen. He then added, 'You know what cuckoos do, don't you? They throw all the babies out of the nest and put their own babies in.' He then continued, 'Their Mum doesn't come to save them. She isn't there and she doesn't care what happens to her children.'

In these three projective techniques, Joseph presented much of his feelings that were creating for him anxiety for which his only outlet was soiling and aggressive behaviour. Joseph completely denied any idea of his mother's consistency of affection for him, of which she herself firmly believed he was aware and which she thought he reciprocated.

## The Use of the ORT with Adolescents

The Object Relations Technique is a particularly delightful one to use with adolescents, who generally seem to find it at least acceptable, and often attractive.

The basic form of the technique is again a story telling one. The material consists of 13 cards in three series, each depicting a one-person, a two-person, a three-person and a group situation. The series vary in their texture and in the amount of detail included. Thus the A series is in soft texture, with very light shading and indefinite detail. The B series has much darker shading and stronger contrasts, and the C series introduces colour and provides much more realistic settings.

The cards combine two of the main threads in the development of projective material, that of the picture-story type, and that of the Rorschach, which also uses colour and texture as important elements.

Whilst some adolescents are willing to talk, and indeed are articulate and forceful in what they have to say, others are very difficult to draw into conversation. Either way the age group as a whole is often notoriously liable to play down its most pressing problems. Many young people dislike direct questioning, as, of course, do many adults, and yet are affected by underlying concerns. Many of these are very common, and indeed almost inevitable.

Conflicts arise at home around growing independence, about friendships and through the need to test out opinions and values in argument. At school the problems may centre on academic success or failure, examinations, career choices, relationships to teachers and attempts at rebelliousness. The development of the adolescent's self-image is throughout a central preoccupation.

Sandra was a 15 year old who was referred as possibly 'dyslexic'. She described herself as having a spelling and writing problem which she feared would spoil her chances of success in her GCE 'O' levels. This had become increasingly worrying to her and her teachers saw her as spoiling her peformance by her slowness, so that 'O' levels were indeed at risk, although her basic ability had not been questioned.

Tests showed her to have a very high level of vocabulary, to do extremely well in all types of verbal reasoning and in no respect did she fall below the 90th percentile for her age except when she was aware of having to work at speed. Her reading was fluent and an inspection of her spelling errors revealed that these were linked to her use of a very large vocabulary with unusual and complex phonic combinations rather than to anything which might be labelled dyslexic.

Some of Sandra's teachers described her as careless and the psychologist's refusal to agree to a diagnosis of dyslexia seemed to leave her with no defence to fall back on. Her anxiety was very high and she readily agreed that tension was a problem.

Her efforts at relaxation were not at all successful, although she had tried exercises. She agreed that she might be lacking in confidence and seemed to accept that the label 'dyslexic' might in the end only add to her poor view of herself. Whilst it was clear that her problems were still unresolved the discussions were apparently grinding to a halt.

With Sandra's agreement that the ORT might help us both to a better understanding of her as a person, she spent the next few weeks, on the basis of one session a week, responding to the ORT cards and discussing the stories she told and their outcomes.

Her stories demonstrated how creatively imaginative she could be. She enjoyed the cards and gave her stories fluently and easily. She often employed very beautiful metaphors, her characters were full of feeling and her ability to respond to the cards was sensitive and her stories quite elegant. Nevertheless she betrayed concern that words, however well used, could never really convey proper meaning. For example, in her very first story a man cannot find the words to say what he feels until he discovers an old photograph which says it all for him. In other stories, sitting around discussing things is presented as leading nowhere and people try to obtain meaning from beautiful art or gardens.

Fears of stupidity and madness arise, characters feel that they have made a fool of themselves or that they are going mad. Sometimes an ending was contrived which made fun of fears of the dark or of ghosts, resolved then by some such ending as siblings teasing or playing jokes on each other. Comfort was also sought, after some more or less fearful or exciting experience in the stories.

This might take the form of getting home for tea and hot scones, or seeking out some other familiar setting. In one very intensely expressed story an old man anticipated grief that his perfect child, clever and attractive, would be killed in a coming war. In other ways too there was a rather dreamy sense of loss, of people and opportunities.

In deciding which of these themes could be explored, initially it seemed important to remain linked to the problem that had first brought Sandra. Therefore we talked about the difficulties her characters had in expressing themselves in words, when she herself was so clearly skilful, and gifted even, in this respect. Sandra explained how she knew she was good with words, always striving in fact to increase her vocabulary as we had already discovered. On the other hand she also rather despised them as somehow artificial, unnatural. This conflict between seeking on the one hand to control the world by words, whilst on the other wanting to be in touch with something primitive and exciting, which would however be out of control, led us into looking at the nature of her ambition.

Only after some time did the link between her ambition and her father become open enough to be related to the perfect child story. Father's teasing was revealed as something which could make Sandra feel ugly and stupid, although there was no suggestion that this was intended.

Her own wish to be the perfect daughter was tested out against her father's opinion of her, which could never be good enough to satisfy her.

We talked of the despair which ambition can bring, useful though it is in pressing one forward. Sandra's way of controlling feelings by gently mocking them was raised in connection with the characters in her stories and she acknowledged that she could never allow herself to cry. She talked more openly of how much she minded about things ending, how she was unable to cope with the feeling that she would not see someone again.

The final session was calm and thoughtful. Sandra said she trusted herself more. She was still afraid of being trivial, rebutting anything she felt had been silly in what she had said, but she was more willing to take a risk in a relationship in the interests of being true to herself. She was also more willing to make allowances for others. She commented also on how much fathers mean to their daughters and this was discussed in a general way.

Throughout Sandra was not pressed to reveal more of her

family, nor were interpretations offered of her relationships at home. The themes raised were always drawn from her stories and were not in the first place presented as giving a direct picture of herself. Nevertheless Sandra often made such links and by the end it seems that she did indeed know herself better. She sat her exams successfully some few months later.

## Conclusion

The children who appear in this chapter are each, of course, unique and their responses can only illustrate the various ways in which projective techniques can help to illuminate their anxieties and the pressures they experience. Not only does the material obtained help in recognising the extent of such anxieties, it may in itself provide a basis for discussion with the children themselves, thus increasing their own understanding and helping them to bring such worries under conscious control.

## References

1. Francis-Williams, Jessie, *Rorschach with Children* (Pergamon Press, Oxford, 1968).

2. Alcock, Theodora, *The Rorschach in Practice* (Tavistock Publications, London, 1963).

3. Phillipson, H., *The Object Relations Technique* (Tavistock Publications, London, 1955).

4. Phillipson, H., *A Short Introduction to the Object Relations Technique* (N.F.E.R., Windsor, Berkshire, 1973).

5. Abt, L. E., 'A Theory of Projective Psychology' in L. E. Abt and L. Bellack (eds), *Projective Psychology*, Part 1. *The Theoretical Foundations of Projective Psychology* (Alfred A. Knopf, New York, 1950).

6. Bruner, J. S., 'Personality Dynamics and the Process of Perceiving' in R. R. Blake and G. V. Ramsay (eds), *Perception, an Approach to Personality* (Ronald Press, New York, 1951).

7. Lowenfeld, M., 'The World Pictures of Children: a Method of Recording and Studying Them', *British Journal of Medical Psychology*, **18** (1939), pp. 65–101.

8. Moore, Terence and Ucko, L. E., 'Four to Six, Constructiveness and Conflict in Meeting Doll Play Problems, *Journal of Child Psychology and Psychiatry*, **2** (1961), pp. 21–47.

9. Bellak, L. and Bellak, S., *The Thematic Apperception Test and the Children's Apperception Test in Clinical Use* (Grune and Stratton, New York, 1957).

10. Ames, L. B., Learned, J., Metraux, R. W. and Walker, R. N., *Child Rorschach Responses* (Hoeber-Harper, New York, 1952).

11. Ames, L. B., Metraux, R. W. and Walker, R. N., *Adolescent Rorschach Responses* (Hoeber-Harper, New York, 1959).

12. Halpern, Florence, *A Clinical Approach to Children's Rorschachs* (Grune and Stratton, New York, 1953).

13. Rabin, Albert L. and Haworth, Mary R. (eds), *Projective Techniques with Children* (Grune and Stratton, New York, 1960).

14. Pickford, R. W., *Pickford Projective Pictures* (Tavistock Publications, London, 1963).

15. Klopfer, B. *et al.*, *Developments in the Rorschach Technique* (Harrap, London, vol. 1 1954, vol. 2 1956).

16. Exner, J. E., *The Rorschach: A Comprehensive System* (John Wiley and Sons, New York, 1974).

17. Anthony, E. J. and Bene, E., 'A Technique for the Objective Assessment of the Child's Family Relationships', *Journal of Mental Science*, **2** (1957), pp. 541–55.

# 5 ANXIETY IN CHILDREN: A CROSS-CULTURAL PERSPECTIVE

Vaman G. Lokare

## Introduction

As a distinct variety of species we all belong to the same species of
*Homo sapiens*. Though groups of people living in different parts of
the world tend to differ from one another in some inherited
physical characteristics, the biological differences that enable us to
classify the human species into races are superficial ones. Besides,
human beings are able to interbreed and interbreeding in humans
has occurred frequently over thousands of years, and hence the
concept of 'pure race' is a myth. Culture, on the other hand, could
mean mental training and development, refinement or civilisation
and the upbringing of children.

Since the last war there has been increasing interest in cross-
cultural problems. There are obviously many reasons for this.
Perhaps one is the situation where the individual has difficulty
forming and maintaining his own cultural identity, which is nowadays to be seen in many European countries with 'guest workers'
and in Britain with the settlers from the commonwealth countries
who form minority groups. Even countries like the USA are not
free from problems of cultural identity with their attendant
anxieties and consequences. Members of minority cultural groups
often identify themselves with the dominant majority and in their
attempts to assimilate in the culture, they sometimes change names,
religion and try actively to reject and forget old customs, language,
life-style etc. Individuals may be seen to vacillate between two
cultures, who until now have lived in some degree of isolation, but
due to better communications have increased contacts with the
surrounding majority, as in the case of Eskimos and Laps. Surely
this struggle with identity creates feelings of insecurity leading to
anxieties and worries which are reflected as feelings of uncertainty
and insufficiency in bringing up one's children, giving them rules,
norms and traditions to follow. Often this kind of struggle to attain
cultural identity gets mixed up with ethnic identity and becomes

entangled in problems of discrimination. Hence I start with an attempt to define the variables, culture and anxiety, the two variables with which this chapter is mainly concerned.

## Culture and Anxiety

The human child is born into a society made up of a group of people dependent upon one another, who have developed patterns of behaviour essential for the survival of the group. Hence it is important for every individual child to learn the ready-made pattern of behaviour and thinking that exists in society and which is transmitted from generation to generation within a continuing society, as this is essential for the individual's survival as the society develops. These prescribed patterns of behaviour, customs, beliefs, etc., make up a large aspect of what is meant by culture. As McKeachie and Doyle[1] put it 'we consider culture to be the patterns of behaving and thinking and products of behaviour that are transferred from generation to generation within any continuing society.'

The behaviour and attitudes of an individual are regarded as normal or abnormal according to the cultural milieu in which the behaviour takes place. However, most societies are not rigid taskmasters and allow reasonable latitude for individuality of expression. Radical aberrations that create turmoil in the individual of those about him are usually looked upon as abnormal behaviours, and/or evidence of an abnormal personality. Horney[2] describes anxiety as a feeling of hopelessness in a potentially hostile world. This, according to her, develops out of the interplay between feelings of anxiety and hostility stirred up by rejecting parental attitudes and is the cause of neurosis. She suggests that many reactions which we look upon as being neurotic in one culture are considered quite normal in another, and also that many conflicts developed by the individual mirror the contradictions in the society.

Mead[3] says that culture

is the term applied to the total shared learning behaviour of a society or a subgroup so we may speak of 'a culture' using the term for a whole, or for an item of behaviour as 'cultural', as referring this item to the whole. The moral situation on which the anthropoligical aspect of culture is based, is that of the total learned, shared behaviour of a functional autonomous society that has maintained its existence through a sufficient number of generations, so that each stage of the life span of the individual is included within the system

Gorer[4] extends this to mean that culture is 'primarily mental or psychological, as non-biological learned behaviour ultimately derivable from the nerves and brain cells of the personnel comprising a given society at a given time'. He also says that

cultural behaviour is learned behaviour . . . learning can be divided into two categories: (1) learning situations in which certainly the teacher, and usually the pupil are conscious and can be articulate about what is being taught, and (2) learning that is not articulate or verbalised by the teacher (if there is one) which the teacher may not be conscious of teaching and which may not be imparted or deliberately conceptualised as a total concept.

In fact he sees culture as the result of both kinds of learning.

The term culture in this chapter refers to the more or less organised and relatively persistent patterns of habits, ideas, attitudes, bodies of knowledge, skills and values in a society, which are passed on to the individual, and which the individual imitates, intentionally or unintentionally, as this provides him with a framework within which he learns to function with those who are close to him. Changes may take place over centuries or even within a decade. For Sinha[5] culture is basic to anxiety. This brings us to the question of anxiety and its definition.

Anxiety is a universal experience. It has been described as a form of vigilance which occurs after encountering danger. McDougall[6] says that anxiety is a complex emotion, and is essentially a matter of alertness or watchfulness. According to Freud[7] a child inherits the 'tendency towards objective anxiety'. He also believed that objective anxiety is an expression of the self-preservation instinct and has obvious utility as a defence. Freud's objective anxiety involves a traumatic factor, and he talks of primary and secondary objective anxiety. Traumatic factors such as the birth trauma are involved in the occurrence of primary objective anxiety, while the secondary objective anxiety is elicited by the likelihood of the occurrence of a traumatic event. Judging from other accounts[8–10] this seems to be the present-day psychoanalytical position. Still remaining within the psychoanalytical realm, anxiety may be conceived of as a 'conscious danger signal associated, not only with an external danger, but also with unconscious contents and motivations, the conscious elaboration of which is inhibited or defended against, because such elaboration would place the individual in even more dangers in relation to the external world'.[11] Drever[12] defines anxiety as 'a most prominent component characteristic of various nervous and mental disorders'. Anxiety is defined by May[13] as 'the apprehension cued off by a threat to some value which the individual holds essential to his existence as a personality'.

Anxiety could also be defined as an innate capacity of an organism to react and it has some inherited neurophysiological concomitants and 'the particular forms which this capacity to react to threats will assume in a given individual is conditioned by the nature of the threats (environment) and by how the individual has learned to deal with them (past and present experience)'.[13] According to Gray's[14] concept of anxiety at the psychological level, it is an internal state which is entered upon receipt of stimuli associated with punishment or frustrative or novel stimuli: whose behavioural effects consist of inhibition of ongoing behaviour, heightened arousal and heightened attention to environmental stimuli, especially novel ones, and whose function is to enable the organism to decide whether or not the changed circumstances require an alteration of existing behaviour patterns. At the physiological level, it consists of activity in the dorsal ascending noradrenergic bundle (DANB) septohippocampal system (SHS). This definition suggests that there is a strong influence of upbringing social and cultural learning on anxieties in an individual.

In recent years psychologists have attempted to relate the concept of anxiety to learning theories. Both learning theorists and psychoanalysts reflect a somewhat deterministic view of behaviour as they deal with plans and goals as products of the learning histories of individuals. However, while the psychoanalyst is preoccupied with the explanation of deviant behaviour and makes no clear-cut distinction between maturation and socialisation in learning, learning theories emphasise carefully controlled experiments to test specific hypotheses about how socialisation influences personality, and apply the results of such experiments to the area of psychopathology.

Mowrer[15] says that anxiety comes from the individual's 'acts which he has committed but wishes he had not. It is, in other words, a guilt theory of anxiety rather than an impulse theory'. Mowrer also thinks that the only difference between Pavlov and Freud is that the former thought that the danger signal (conditioned stimulis) elicits the same reaction as that previously produced by the actual trauma (stimulus substitution), whereas the latter thought that a danger signal may produce any one of that infinite variety of possible reactions that are unlike those reactions to the original trauma. In other words, this is recasting Freud's theory of anxiety in stimulus-response (SR) terminology. It was this that led Mowrer to develop a theory including fear as a drive, and fear reduction as reinforcement,[16] which he later tested. He found that anxiety reduction was positively correlated with learning.

Miller and Dollard[17] talk of anxiety in terms of its drive properties and believe that anxiety is one of the major sources of human motivation. They think drive is innate and what is acquired is the tendency of a previously neutral stimulus to elicit the drive. In fact, it is the association between the stimulus and drive that has been acquired. To test these hypotheses derived from learning theory Taylor[18] starts from Hull's[19] basic assumption that the excitatory potential (E) determining the strength of a response is a multiplicative function of a learning factor H and a generalised drive factor D, i.e. $E = H \times D$. He assumes that the drive level D is a function of the magnitude or strength of a hypothetical response in the organism — persistent emotional response in the organism which he calls 'r' (fear or anxiety) and conceives drive due to anxiety as non-specific. A similar approach has also been used by Castenada *et al.*[20] in their work with the Children's Manifest Anxiety Scale.

Sarason and Mandler[21] view anxiety as being situation-specific, and aroused in an achievement situation. This they call 'test anxiety'. They emphasise anxiety as a drive stimulus (SD):

anxiety drive which is a function of anxiety reactions, previously learned as responses to stimuli present in the testing situation. Anxiety is here considered as a response-produced stimulus with the function of characteristics of drives as discussed by Miller and Dollard (1941) anxiety reactions are generalised from previous experience in the testing situation.[21]

In terms of the Yerkes-Dodson principle[22] then it would seem to follow Pavlov's laws; the law of strength and the law of trans-marginal inhibition. The former assert that the response strength is proportional to the strength of the stimulus, and the latter, that there is a point of maximum response beyond which any further increase in strength of the stimulus leads to a lessening of response.

In terms of the Yerkes-Dodson principle[22] the relationship between a drive and learning is curvilinear, and is referred to as the inverted-U relation between drive and performance. There is an optimal level of drive for each kind of task which energises the individual and helps to improve performance. While too low a drive, below the optimal level, may produce insufficient motivation, and may be inadequate to improve performance, too high a level of drive exceeding the optimal for a given task may interfere with the learning processes, prove to be disruptive and even lead to maladaptive responses.[23-25] Further, one also has to consider seriously the results of applying the second half of the Yerkes-Dodson Law which says that the relationship between drive and performance is a function of task complexity in that for very simple tasks the optimal level is high, while very difficult tasks have a low optimal drive level. It would therefore follow that the drive level that facilitates performance on a simple task, may disrupt it when the task is more complex and difficult.

If we add to these suggestions the idea that a heightened drive state (anxiety) is linked with a number of previously learned response tendencies, often emotional in nature and even irrelevant to the task in hand, and which disrupt performance by competing with the right response,[21,26] then we reach a situation well described by Gwynne Jones.[27] 'When the correct response is based on relatively weak habit strength, increased drive is deleterious in that the stronger inaccurate tendencies gain relatively more excitatory potential, and have therefore an enhanced probability of evocation.' Here we can add one more controversial, but widely used definition, of anxiety labelled as emotionality, neuroticism or instability which is one part of a two-dimensional system of personality description[28] and which claims to have strong hereditary basis and yet interlocks with certain social and psychiatric methods of classification.[29]

By now it should be obvious that though the number of possible definitions of anxiety is unlimited, all take their origins from some theoretical orientation and hence to a certain extent have abstract contents that often fulfil operational criteria. Anxiety here is considered as a complex concept with respect to its origin, its behavioural effects, and its interindividual differences. It is generally accompanied by some psychosomatic changes, e.g. increases in perspiration, heart-rate, etc. While acting in accord with reality it could be considered as essential and even beneficial, disproportionate anxiety could be a handicap and may even lead to psychopathological conditions. However, all these definitions could be classed under either one or both of the classifications, viz. (1) habitual innate or trait anxiety with possible heredity basis, and (2) situation-produced anxiety on undifferentiated groups of subjects.

The definitions that fall strictly within the first classification emphasise the heredity nature of anxiety and imply a possible (so-called) racial difference in anxiety. The definitions that fall totally within the second classification suggest strong cultural and sub-cultural limitations and expose anxiety to the total mercy of environmental effect in terms of upbringing and education. Some data based on tests claiming to measure general level of anxiety, manifest anxiety, test anxiety and neuroticism are presented here and discussed in the following pages.

**Sex Differences**

A cursory glance at Table 5.1 shows that girls score higher than boys on all anxiety scales, irrespective of the theoretical orientation on which these tests are constructed. One could interpret this to mean that girls are more anxious than boys, and they feel anxiety in a wider variety of situations and that they also feel it more intensively than boys.

One could say that the reasons for the marked differences in anxiety scores between girls and boys is due to the fact that is is easier for girls to admit to anxiety. It means that the differences in the anxiety scores between girls and boys do not reflect an innate difference, but are only a measure of differences in their attitude to admitting to anxiety. Kapoor suggests that the observed sex differences in psychological characteristics are mainly traceable to environmental factors rather than any innate tendencies that are sex-linked. Talking of environmental factors, cultural factors make boys more defensive in admitting anxiety because in the cultures

Table 5.1: Mean Scores for Various Tests on Different Population Samples

| Test | English Children | | American Children | | Indian Children |
|---|---|---|---|---|---|
| | White | Non-white | White | Negro | |
| General Anxiety Scale for Children (GASC) | 11.50[11] to 13.02[31]<br>girls 13.23<br>boys 9.31 | | 12.00[11] | | 19.85[32]<br>girls 20.84<br>boys 18.92 |
| Test Anxiety Scale for Children (TASC) | 10.01[11] to 10.76[31]<br>girls 16.97<br>boys 9.10 | | 7.00[11] | | 16.64[32] |
| Children's Anxiety Scale (CMAS) | girls 20.09 to 21.22[36]<br>boys 16.26 to 18.46[36] | | girls 13.71[33] to 20.75[34]<br>boys 14.61[33] to 17.2[35] | girls 20.75<br>boys 16.59 | |
| Lokare's Modified Junior Maudsley Personality Inventory (LMJMPI) | girls 8.30<br>boys 7.38[25] | girls 8.81<br>boys 7.87 | | | girls 8.95<br>boys 8.88 |

under study they are supposed to be brave. Sarason's[11,21] own alternative explanation as to why boys are more defensive in admitting anxiety implies that the answer may lie in the contents of the GASC itself, as it refers to fears and bodily injuries, etc., which he says boys are naturally likely to be less willing to admit. This cannot be said of the scores of the LMJMPI, as there is no such obvious bias of the contents of the test. It is felt, however, that at the present state of knowledge it is not possible either positively to admit or deny a real sex difference in anxiety. From this one could also jump to the conclusion that anxiety is totally sex-linked and in that sense genetically determined. This would, however, make it difficult to find an acceptable explanation to the differences found between anxiety scores of girls on GASC, TASC and CMAS, tests on Indian, English, American white and American negro girls, and differences between the scores of boys belonging to these various groups. Any attempt to find an explanation in terms of purely hereditary nature of anxiety and to attribute these differences in scores on anxiety to racial differences would create further complications.

First, the mean scores on the GASC for anxious English children in the Sarason *et al.*[11] study is lower than that for the America white children, though not significantly so, but it differs significantly from that reported by Pringle and Cox[31] for English children, and the figures for Indian children in the Nijhawan[32] study.

Second, Sarason's own study[11] shows that the mean score for American white children on the TASC is significantly lower than for English white children, and this is borne out by Pringle and Cox's[31] figures as well. TASC mean scores on Indian children[32] are also significantly higher than those for the American as well as the English children.

Third, the figures for the CMAS scores show a significant difference between those reported by Levitt,[33] Palermo[34] and Rie,[35] between groups of American white children. Again, the scores on the CMAS for English children reported by Colman *et al.*[36] and for American negro children reported by Palermo[34] are both significantly higher than those reported by Levitt[33] for the American white children. However, they do not differ significantly from those reported by Rie[35] and Palermo.[34] It is also obvious that the mean scores, depending on the particular sample may overlap across various racial and cultural groups and also may differ significantly between them.

Lastly, in the LMJMPI scores where anxiety is defined in terms of neuroticism, there is no significant difference in the scores of either girls or boys belonging to various samples, and this is so regardless of their membership of any racial or cultural group.

On the one hand, therefore, it looks as though these differences in anxiety scores relate at least partly to a complex and peculiar combination of differences in race, culture, education and upbringing. On the other hand differences in the anxiety scores could be chance differences due to sampling error or the size of the samples being too small to test the hypothesis. Again, it could reflect the rigidity or the inadequacy of the theoretical orientation and the structure of each one of these tests. Once again of the tests studied LMJPMI[23-25] fails to show significant differences in the scores of children belonging to different racial and cultural groups. This test defines anxiety in terms of neuroticism and hence strongly suggests that there are no racial or cultural differences in anxiety level in school children, but on the other hand, it would also suggest that possibly the test measured a particular aspect or a special feature of anxiety which is uniformly distributed among all the members of the human species. It would also appear that this aspect is not more than marginally, and only insignificantly influenced by differences in culture, education or upbringing. This is borne out by Eysenck's[37] studies with adults where he reports no significant differences in the neuroticism scores for various samples of the American as well as the English population.

**Age Variation**

Literature is full of studies which report age differences in anxiety. Theorising with psychoanalytical as well as learning theory approaches from the time the child starts appraising its relationship with its parents and begins to react to the impact of evaluative quality of their behaviour, it should show an upward trend in the development of anxiety. Sarason[38] and Thompson[39] in their studies with TASC report that anxiety increased with age. Eysenck[40] reported a similar trend in that girls became more unstable with increasing age, but this applied to boys of only seven or eight years of age. Lokare[25] also reported similar trends, but only in boys of eight, nine and ten years of age. This would in general support Freud's theory according to which as the ego matures there is an increase in the ability to judge events and to anticipate the future.

With this comes a more realistic perception of danger and consequently an increase in anxiety. Like Sullivan[41] one can describe fear as self-protective reaction to a painful or novel situation and anxiety as a product of education. This restated could mean fear is an unconditioned (unlearned) response to a potentially harmful stimulus (usually direct pain, etc.) while anxiety is a conditioned fear response to a new situation. This is further illustrated by the fact[42] that the fears observed in infants are related to transient but specific stimuli (e.g. loud noises, dropping, strange people, etc.); but as the child grows older the fears are replaced by anxieties of an anticipatory or imaginary character (darkness, ghosts, being bad). This would also support the theory that anxiety is learned and not inherited. Therefore, it would seem to follow that to look for purely racial and genetic differences in anxiety would not be a very rewarding exercise, as whatever differences are found could all have a strong cultural and educational stamp in terms of learnt behaviour. Nijhawan,[32] however, in a study of GASC and TASC, and Angelino *et al.*[43] in their study of situation anxiety reported that anxiety is somewhat negatively related to age. In their studies with CMAS both Palermo[34] and Colman *et al.*[36] reported that there is some indication of an inverse relationship between age and anxiety. Eysenck[40] reported a similar trend in boys from nine years upwards, in her studies with the Junior Eysenck Personality Inventory. Lokare[25] also reported a similar trend in boys of ten years upwards and girls from eight years upwards. This suggests a possible strong influence of developmental factors related to maturation and growth in terms of psychophysiological mechanisms, rather than purely in terms of the maturation of the ego or solely as the result of learning theories.

Besides, there is evidence to suggest that the basic tendency to react with anxiety diminishes, though only slightly, with very large increases in age, even in adults.[28] All this goes to imply that anxiety is a complex concept.

### Socio-economic Status

The role played by socio-economic level in the emotional adjustment of the individual is still little understood. Opinions differ among authors on the issue of the relationship between socio-economic status and anxiety. Brown[44] states that neuroticism does not predominate in any social or cultural group. However, in a later study[45] he reports that differences in emotional stability are not a function of either race or locale, but is closely related to socio-economic level. Springer,[46] using Brown's Personality Inventory for Children and the Haggarty and Olson-Wickman Behaviour Rating Schedule which is closely related to the general social status of the individual and the Barr-Scale of Occupational Status of Fathers also arrived at the conclusion that emotional stability is closely related to the status of the individual child. Sarason *et al.*[11] found that Milford children coming from lower socio-economic status families scored higher than the Greenwich children belonging to upper-class families. Heywood and Dobbs[47] report that children from low socio-economic status groups scored higher on the CMAS than the children from high socio-economic status. Durrett[48] in his study on an Indian sample of Marathi-speaking children, reported a tendency for middle-class income children to score higher on the CMAS than the children belonging to the lower income families, though the differences were not significant. Nijhawan[32] in her study with Indian children reported that the children of lower socio-economic class exhibited significantly higher anxiety than the upper-class children on both the GASC and the TASC. There is a striking similarity between some of her figures for upper-class Indian children and the figures for Western children reported by various authors. At this stage, if we take another look at the figures in Table 11.1, some seemingly obvious explanations for the differences in anxiety scores come to mind. In addition to the racial and cultural differences between the various groups of children, there are also differences in their socio-economic status which could be responsible for the differences. Two of the many studies on adults that support this view are those of Dahlstrom and Welsh[49] on the American sample, and Joshi and Singh[50] on the Indian sample.

Here again, like Becker[51] one looks at self-esteem as a function for avoiding anxiety, then the individuals who have failed to develop adequate self-esteem are likely to be anxious individuals. Wilson[52] argues that anxiety proneness leads to feelings of insecurity and poor self-esteem. Therefore low esteem and anxiety must be positively correlated or it is possible that poor self-esteem[53] is mainly anxiety in context (manifest anxiety). Evan-Wong and Bagley's[54] study which found a correlation of $-0.655$ between Castenada Scale measuring manifest anxiety and Coopersmith Scale measuring self-esteem does suggest that it could be so. These findings add a further complication to the already complex problem of a meaningful interpretation of differences in anxiety found between various groups of children, and even groups of adults, for that matter, belonging to different racial groups, minorities and nationalities. It makes the task of even planning comparative studies of racial and cultural differences much more difficult, as it is not easy to find comparable racial and cultural groups without any differences in their socio-economic level and social status. Besides, it would be difficult to estimate the amount of influence exerted on the level of anxiety by socio-economic level and social status, as these are in turn so interdependent with the cultural values and the philosophy of the people who make up the group.

**Educational Achievements**

So far the whole of the discussion on anxiety has centred around group-likenesses and differences. It is time we looked at this from the point of individual differences. Fortunately there seems to be a universal agreement between all the workers, irrespective of their theoretical background and beliefs, in that they all accept that individuals differ in varying degrees. Everyone also agrees that children could be classified as showing high or low or intermediate levels of anxiety, and that in any given cross-section of society the majority always belong to the group who show neither particularly high or low anxiety, irrespective of race or culture. The effects of anxiety as a drive on behaviour have been assessed by studies of experimentally induced anxiety, or by using children who have been found to be high or low in anxiety. Two important issues studied in this way are the relationship of anxiety and educational achievement, and the relationship of anxiety to behavioural adjustment. Sarason *et al.*[11] reported significant negative correlations between anxiety and performance on educational achievement and intelligence tests. Gaudry and Bradshaw[55] found that children with high anxiety score significantly lower in class tests than those with low anxiety. Cox[56] also studied the relationship of anxiety on school assessment marks. He reported that about three-quarters of the medium anxiety group are in the top half of the class, as compared with approximately half of the low-anxiety group and less than one-third of the high-anxiety group. This seems to support

Hebb's[57] theory that the optimal level of motivation for effective performance lies in the middle ranges rather than at the high or low end. One can see how this also supports the formalised Yerkes-Dodson law[22] which states that the relationship between motivation (anxiety) and learning takes the form of the inverted U-shaped curve mentioned earlier. A vast number of studies carried out along these lines so far show that anxiety tends to impair children's problem-solving ability. The most consistent general findings so far are that high anxiety is associated with relatively low performance at both school and university level. This is irrespective of the type of test used for measuring anxiety, and the varieties of measures of academic achievements used. Studies so far have also indicated that high-anxious children have more difficulty with complex learning tasks than low-anxious children, because of the arousal of competing responses, more of which are raised to threshold level for the high-anxious child. However, the opposite is true for simple learning situations where the scope of possible responses is restricted. Low anxiety may produce insufficient motivation which may be inadequate to improve performance and too high anxiety may increase drive and motivation to a level that exceeds the optimum for a given task and thus interferes with the learning process and even leads to maladaptive responses. In other words, the differences between the highly anxious and low-anxious children are particularly marked when the tasks are difficult or require creative solutions or when the test situation is a threatening one. A classroom situation could become more threatening under various conditions, e.g. tests and examinations, the presence or absence of a person other than the tester,[58] the sex and the membership of racial or cultural group of the tester, etc.

**General Guidelines and Implications**

In the classroom and in day-to-day life, one often comes across children with varying degrees of adjustment problems, some of whom may be diagnosed as suffering from neurotic illness. Though a large number of such children are highly anxious, one also finds individuals who do not show high anxiety. It is also a fact that there are numerous individuals who are reasonably well adjusted and yet show high anxiety. One of the possible explanations could be that in the former case the stresses and strains were perhaps too great and beyond the individual's capacity to cope with, while in the latter case possibly the individual was not exposed to stresses and strains beyond the limits of his capacity to cope. In other words, it is apparent that apart from anxiety, the circumstances and the situations play quite an important part in bringing about the resultant behaviour, whether normal or abnormal. Anxiety which is associated with a state of apprehension, worry, sense of insecurity and the need for reassurance is largely anticipatory. Yet, without some degree of anxiety in accord with reality, an individual would be without concern, even for events and things that are essential for survival and welfare.[59] Morbid anxiety, however, overwhelms the individual and leads to a host of psychological problems.

All this goes to suggest that anxiety, which is a universal experience, is also a most important emotion from the teacher's and therapist's point of view because of its effect on learning, achievement and adjustment. Anxiety is also a complex concept and it involves an intricate and extremely complex relationship between other personality variables, biological inherited characteristics, cultural influences, the impact of education and the effects of different patterns of upbringing. One must remember therefore not to attribute specific (pathological) levels of anxiety to every member of a cultural group as this would amount to assuming trans-situational generality of anxiety, relative immutability of the behaviour concerned in new situations (e.g. after cultural dislocation) and early origins with fixed limitations during the life cycle of an individual. Forgetting this caution one could easily take behaviours to be parts of a specific cultural orientation without allowing scope for specific learned isolated reaction tendencies. Hence, in making extra special arrangements for the children of the minority group, one should bear in mind the possible risks of engendering feelings of inferiority, helplessness and insecurity in them while fostering prejudices and stereotyping and the like in teachers, therapists and children of the minority group.[59] In this way, unless one is extremely careful, things may go from bad to worse. Our ability to identify the individual anxious child and the environmental stress or stresses that trigger off this anxiety, together with increased knowledge of handling, is likely to prove to be of greater practical value when a particular child develops a problem rather than concentrating on general characteristics and stereotyping.

# References

1. McKeachie, W. J. and Doyle, C. L., *Psychology* (Addison Wesley Publishing Co. Inc., Reading, Mass., 1966).

2. Horney, K., *The Neurotic Personality of Our Time* (Norton, New York, 1937).

3. Mead, M., 'Study of Culture at a Distance', in Mead and Me'traux (eds), *Study of Culture at a Distance* (The University of Chicago Press, Ill., 1953).

4. Gorer, G., 'National Character: Theory and Practice', in *The Study of Culture at a Distance* (eds Mead and Me'traux) (The University of Chicago Press, Chicago, 1953).

5. Sinha, D., 'Cultural Factors in the Emergence of Anxiety', *Eastern Anthropologist, 15* (1962) pp. 21–37.

6. McDougall, W., *An Introduction to Social Psychology* (Methuen, London, 1908).

7. Freud, S., *The Problem of Anxiety* (Translated by Bunker, H. A., American edn) (W. W. Norton and Co. Inc., New York, 1936).

8. Hoch, P. and Zubin, J., *Anxiety* (Grune and Stratton, New York, 1950).

9. Rosenberg, E., 'Anxiety and the Capacity to Bear it', *International Journal of Psycho-Analysis, 30* (1949), pp. 1–12.

10. Roycroft, C., *Anxiety and Neurosis* (Allen Lane, The Penguin Press, London, 1968).

11. Sarason, S. B., Davidson, K. S., Lighthall, F. F., Waite, R. R. and Ruebush, B. K., *Anxiety in Elementary School Children: a Report of Research* (J. Wiley and Sons Inc., New York, 1960).

12. Drever, J., *A Dictionary of Psychology* (Penguin, Harmondsworth, London, 1958).

13. May, R., *The Meaning of Anxiety* (Ronald Press, New York, 1950).

14. Gray, J. A., 'The Neuropsychology of Anxiety', *British Journal of Psychology, 69* (1978), p. 417.

15. Mowrer, O. H., *Learning Theory and Personality Dynamics* (The Ronald Press Co., New York, 1950).

16. Mowrer, O. H., 'A Stimulus-Response Analysis of Anxiety and its Role as a Reinforcing Agent', *Psychological Review, 46* (1939), pp. 553–65.

17. Miller, N. E. and Dollard, J., *Social Learning and Imitation* (Yale University Press, New Haven, Connecticut, 1941).

18. Taylor, J. A., 'Drive Theory and Manifest Anxiety', *Psychology Bulletin, 53* (1956), pp. 303–20.

19. Hull, C. L., *Principles of Behaviour* (Appleton Century Crofts, New York, 1943).

20. Castenada, A., McCandless, B. R. and Palermo, D. S., 'The Children's Form of the Manifest Anxiety Scale', *Child Development, 27* (1956), pp. 317–26.

21. Sarason, S. B. and Mandler, G., 'Some Correlates of Test Anxiety', *Journal of Abnormal Social Psychology, 47*, (1952), pp. 810–16.

22. Yerkes, R. M. and Dodson, J. D., 'The Relation of Strength of Stimulus to Rapidity of Habit-formation', *Journal of Comparative Neurology and Psychology, 18* (1908), pp. 459–82.

23. Lokare, V. G. 'The Clinical Application of a Children's Personality Inventory', *Proceedings of the Sixth International Congress on Psychology and Psychiatry*, Edinburgh.

24. Lokare, V. G., 'The Application of the Lokare's Modified Junior Maudsley Personality Inventory with Particular Reference to 8–12 Year Old Children', *Journal of Child Psychology and Psychiatry, 13* (1972), pp. 37–46.

25. Lokare, V. G., Neuroticism and Extraversion in Children as Measured by the Lokare's Modified Junior Maudsley Personality Inventory. M. Phil. Thesis (1972).

26. Child, I. L., 'Personality', *Annual Reviews of Psychology, 5* (1954), pp. 149–70.

27. Jones, Gwynne, 'Learning and Abnormal Behaviour', in Eysenck (ed.), *Handbook of Abnormal Psychology* (Pitman, London, 1960).

28. Eysenck, H. J., *The Structure of Human Personality* (Methuen, London, 1953).

29. Eysenck, H. J., *The Biological Basis of Personality* (Thomas, Springfield, Ill., 1967).

30. Kapoor, S. D., 'Personality Differences Between the Sexes', *Psychology Studies, 9* (1964), pp. 124–32.

31. Pringle, M. L. K. and Cox, J., 'The Influence of Schooling and Sex on Test and General Anxiety as Measured by Sarason's Scales', *Journal of Child Psychology and Psychiatry, 4* (1963), pp. 157–65.

32. Nijhawan, H. K., *Anxiety in School Children* (Wiley, Eastern Private Ltd, New Delhi, 1972).

33. Levitt, E. E., 'Ecological Differences in Performance on the CMAS, *Psychology Reports, 3* (1957), pp. 281–6.

34. Palermo, D. S., 'Racial Comparisons and Additional Normative Data on the Children's Manifest Anxiety Scale', *Childhood Development, 30* (1959), pp. 53–7.

35. Rie, H. E., 'An Exploratory Study of the CMAS Lie Scale', *Child Development, 34* (1963), pp. 1003–17.

36. Colman, S. W., Mackay, D. and Fidell, B., 'English Normative Data on the Children's Manifest Anxiety Scale', *British Journal of Social and Clinical Psychology, 2* (1972), pp. 85–7.

37. Eysenck, H. J., *Manual of the Maudsley Personality Inventory* (University of London Press, London, 1959).

38. Sarason, S. B., 'Test Anxiety', *Journal of the National Education Association, 48* (1959), pp. 26–7.

39. Thompson, G. G., *Child Psychology* (Times of India Press, Bombay, 1965).

40. Eysenck, S. B. G., *Manual of the Junior Eysenck Personality Inventory* (University of London Press, London, 1965).

41. Sullivan, H. S., *Clinical Studies in Psychiatry* (Norton, New York, 1956).

42. Valentine, W. L., *Experimental Foundations of General Psychology* (Rinehart, New York, 1941).

43. Angelino, H., Dollin, J. and Mech, E. V., 'Trends in the "Fears and Worries" of School Children as Revealed to Socio-economic Status and Age', *Journal of General Psychology, 89* (1956), pp. 263–76.

44. Brown, F. A., 'A Psychoneurotic Inventory for Children Between Nine and Fourteen Years of Age', *Journal of Applied Psychology, 19* (1934), pp. 566–77.

45. Brown, F. A., 'A Comparative Study of the Influence of Race and Locale upon Emotional Stability of Children', *Journal of Genetics and Psychology, 49* (1936), pp. 325–42.

46. Springer, N. N., 'The Influence of General Social Status on the Emotional Stability of Children', *Journal of General Psychology, 53* (1938), pp. 321–8.

47. Heywood, H. C. and Dobbs, V., 'Motivation and Anxiety in High School Boys', *Journal of Personality, 32* (1964), pp. 371–9.

48. Durrett, M. A., 'Normative Data on the Children's Manifest Anxiety Scale for Marathi-speaking Indian Children on Different Income Levels', *Indian Journal of Psychology, 40* (1965), pp. 1–6.

49. Dahlstrom, W. G. and Welsh, G. S., *An MMPI Handbook* (Minnesota Press, Minneapolis, 1960).

50. Joshi, M. C. and Singh, B., 'Influence of Socio-economic Background on the Scores of Some MMPI Scales', *Journal of Social Psychology, 70* (1966), pp. 241–425.

51. Becker, E., *The Birth and Death of Meaning* (Penguin Books, London, 1971).

52. Wilson, G., *The Psychology of Conservatism* (Academic Press, London, 1973).

53. Coopersmith, S., *The Antecedants of Self-Esteem* (Freeman, San Francisco, 1967).

54. Evan-Wong, L. and Bagley, C., 'Cognitive Complexity and Self-esteem'. Unpublished study. (Referred to by Bagley C., Verma, G. K., Mallick, K. and Young, L. in *Personality, Self-Esteem* and *Prejudice* (Saxon House, 1979).

55. Gaudry, E. E. and Bradshaw, G. D., 'The Differential Effects of Anxiety on Performance in Progressive and Terminal School Examinations', *Australian Journal of Psychology, 22* (1970), pp. 1–4.

56. Cox, F. N., 'Correlates of General and Test Anxiety in Children', *Australian Journal of Psychology, 12* (1960), pp. 69–77.

57. Hebb, D. O., *A Text Book of Psychology* (Saunders, London, 1958).

58. Cox, F. N., 'Some Relationships Between Test Anxiety Presence or Absence of Male Persons and Boys Performance on a Repetitive Motor Task', *Journal of Experimental Child Psychology, 6* (1968), pp. 11–12.

59. Lokare, V. G., *Therapies in Child and Youth Psychiatry*. vol. 2, Proc. Vth Congress of the Union of European Pedopsychiatrists, Vienna, (1975), pp. 263–8.

# 6 FAMILY DYSFUNCTION AND ANXIETY IN CHILDREN

Philip Barker

Other chapters in this book have looked at anxiety in children mainly from the point of view of the child, and his or her intra-psychic processes. Children however exist as parts of family systems and often a full understanding of a child's anxiety is possible only in the light of an understanding of the family system of which he/she is a part. The point has been made, in Chapter 3, that psychiatric interviews with children must be supplemented by interviews with their parents. This is not simply to obtain information about the child's history, behaviour or symptomatology, but also to gain an understanding of the wider family system. But family assessment, which aims to look at the family system as a whole, comprises very much more than simply interviewing the parents to discuss a child's development and problems. It usually involves at least one interview with the whole family group, which should normally include all members of the current household.

## The Family as a System

A system was defined by von Bertalanffy[1] as 'a complex of inter-acting elements'. Hall and Fagan[2] define a system as 'a set of objects together with the relationships between the objects and between their attributes'. Systems theory can be used to deal with both living and non-living systems; thus it covers physical phenomena and machines as well as biological systems. In dealing with biological, and especially social systems, however, systems theory cannot be applied in a precise mathematical fashion. The more modest term 'systems thinking'[3] is probably better applied to the current state of understanding of family systems. The principal ideas which family therapists have derived from systems theory are:[4]

1. Families (and other social groups) are systems having

properties which are more than the sum of properties of their parts.

2. There are certain general rules which govern the operation of such systems.

3. Every system has a boundary, the properties of which are important in understanding how the system works.

4. Boundaries are semi-permeable.

5. Family systems tend to reach a relatively, but not totally, steady state. Growth and evolution are possible, indeed usual. Change can occur, or be effected, in various ways.

6. Communication and feedback mechanisms between the parts of the system are important in the functioning of the system.

7. Events such as the behaviour of individuals in the family are better understood as examples of *circular causality*, rather than *linear causality*.

8. Family systems, like other open systems, have the property of *equifinality*, that is the same end-point may be reached from a number of starting points.

9. Family systems, like other open systems, appear to have a purpose.

10. Systems are made up of *subsystems* and themselves are parts of *suprasystems*.

In a family the subsystems will consist of various individuals or groups of individuals. There will be boundaries between the various subsystems. Examples are parental, marital or child subsystems. There may be boy and girl subsystems or subsystems consisting of older and younger children. Suprasystems to which families may belong include the extended family, the village, the neighbourhood, the tribe, church communities and so on. These in turn are part of yet larger suprasystems, until we get nations, groups of nations and planet earth itself. The earth in turn of course is part of the solar system which is part of a yet larger celestial system.

Individuals too are composed of subsystems, whether biological, as exemplified in the cardiac, respiratory, endocrine and other bodily systems; or psychological as exemplified by such constructs as the ego, the id and the superego.

Each family system has its own structure and way of functioning. It also has a boundary, marking it off from its surroundings. While living systems have readily identifiable physical boundaries, such as skin or the bark of trees, the boundaries of human social systems are less obviously visible, though equally important. They influence the emotional exchanges, closeness and joint actions of those on either side. When family therapists refer to certain family members as belonging to particular subsystems, they usually mean that there is a high degree of emotional closeness. Thus the boundary between one subsystem and another subsystem will be characterised by restricted emotional interchange, compared with that occurring within the subsystems. Similar considerations apply to the boundaries between subsystems and their suprasystems, and between systems — for example one family group and another.

Family systems are 'open' in that there is interchange, between them and their suprasystems, that is the environment outside. They are not totally open however, and within their boundaries the parts of the system interact in particular ways which tend to remain relatively constant, though change and growth are normally occurring also. This is necessary since in any family developmental changes occur as children are born, grow up, start school, reach adolescence and leave home. The parents are then left with an 'empty nest', and later face retirement.

Circular, as opposed to linear, causality is characteristic of family systems. Thus it is not usually possible to see simple chains of events as when event A causes event B and there are no further repercussions. When this happens the term linear causality is applied. Thus when it starts to rain, a man may put up his umbrella, but putting up the umbrella is not generally believed to have an effect on whether or not it rains. This is therefore a case of linear causality. Circular causality operates when event A leads to event B, which then effects event A, perhaps through the mediation of events C,D,E, and more.

An example of circular causality is the case of a family containing a girl with severe obsessive-compulsive symptoms (see Chapter 3 and also *Basic Child Psychiatry*[5]). Nicole presented with a wide variety of ritualistic behaviours which caused her to take up to two hours to get dressed in the morning. Eating meals was similarly ritualised, Nicole's food having first to be cut up into small pieces, then segregated into different types, then brought up to her mouth and back to the plate three times before Nicole would eat it. The problem seemed to have started, though, with a fear of 'germs'. This began after a talk on hygiene by a nurse at school. The parents tried to reassure Nicole, for example, by cutting a little of her food off and eating it first to show that it was not contaminated by germs. By the time Nicole and her family were seen the parents were busy trying to adapt to Nicole's rituals, and to reassure her about her worries, which in turn intensified the obsessive-compulsive behaviours, perhaps because adapting to the rituals carried the implied message that they were justified. This then caused the parents to increase their efforts to accommodate Nicole. Psychiatric referral occurred when finally Nicole was eating so little that she began rapidly to lose weight. The circular process — a 'positive feedback loop' — had to be broken by having the parents order Nicole to cease her rituals and physically prevent her from carrying them out.

Most circular processes are less dramatic than this and involve mundane, everyday behaviours, which usually reach a 'steady state' and do not escalate as Nicole's symptoms did.

Epstein *et al.*,[6] offer a model of the functioning of family systems. This distinguishes six aspects of family functioning:

1. The family's methods and style of problem solving.
2. The family's communication patterns.
3. The roles of the different family members.
4. The affective responsiveness of family members to each other.
5. The affective involvement of the various family members.
6. The methods of behavioural control used in the family.

For a description of these different aspects of family functioning the reader should refer to the paper by Epstein and his colleagues; a summary is also to be found in *Basic Family Therapy*.[4] In understanding the anxious child, the concept of family members' roles is particularly helpful, though the other aspects are relevant too.

Roles are the habitual patterns of behaviour that the members of a family display. They are also necessary for the carrying out of a family's various functions. Epstein and his colleagues[6] point out that there are *instrumental* and *affective* functions that have to be performed in families. Family functioning can also be broken down into 'necesary' and 'other' family functions. Necessary functions include the provision of physical resources for the family, the nurture and support of family members, the sexual gratification of the marital partners, life skill development and the maintenance and management of the family system. The performance of all these functions requires that particular members play certain specific roles in the family, though who does what may vary from time to time.

'Other' family functions are those which are unique to a family, or at least are not universally necessary. In many 'dysfunctional' families individual members, who are often children, are left performing idiosyncratic and sometimes very difficult roles which may lead to their developing a moderate or even a high level of anxiety. Of course a 'functional' as opposed to a 'dysfunctional', family will operate in such a way that no individual member is unduly stressed by performing the role which the system requires of him/her. (To say that the system requires a person to play a particular role is not strictly correct, and smacks of linear causality. In fact the individual's behaviour in his/her role influences the system as much as the system influences the behaviour, but for the sake of brevity this point will not be emphasised every time an individual's behaviour in relation to the family system is mentioned.)

### Stressful Family Situations

Common stressful family situations are those in which one or more members find themselves playing roles which are difficult for them, and thus anxiety provoking; and those which arise when a family runs into difficulties negotiating a particular developmental stage. Such situations may of course provoke anxiety in adult family members as well as in child members, but this account will focus on the effects on children. Thus anxiety in children may arise in the following situations:

1. The child's role may be too big for the resources available to the child:
   (a) The child may be called upon to be peacemaker between the parents or between other family members. Where there is continuing marital strife it is not uncommon to find that the family system functions in such a way that the child or children are drawn into the conflict in ways which tend to defuse it. They may directly intervene on behalf of one or the other of the warring parties but more

often they try and defuse the conflict by behaving badly in some way. This may enable the parents to unite in dealing with the children's bad behaviour; they are thus diverted from their own disagreements. Such peacekeeping efforts are usually only temporarily, and often only partially, effective and the child may have to redouble his/her efforts to achieve results. If the results sought are not obtained as a result of the child's behaviour this can be disheartening or even anxiety-provoking and depressing to the child. It should be realised however that in most cases the behaviour on the child's part is not part of a conscious effort to be a peacemaker. It is rather an unconsciously triggered automatic reaction to the conflict between the parents.

(b) The child may play the role of mediator between family members, especially the parents. In cases of severe marital conflict this too can often be a bigger role than the child can effectively carry out. Children who function as mediators tend to present the view of one parent to the other one and on some occasions may go repeatedly from one parent to the other to try and patch up differences, rather like an American envoy mediating between Middle Eastern states. In many cases however the child's mediating powers are not adequate for the task required. Thus the child becomes increasingly stressed and anxious. The child's anxiety may be compounded by feelings of guilt arising from the failure to accomplish mediation successfully.

(c) The child may attempt to detour conflict. Thus when one parent is angry with another, or the parent is angry with another child, a child may behave in such a way as to draw the parent's attention to his/her own behaviour, as a way of diverting it from its original objective. Children may try to protect their mothers or their siblings, or sometimes their fathers, in this way. This is somewhat similar to peacemaking, except that the objective is not to improve the relationship between the parents, or other family members, but simply to draw the anger of one member of the family away from its original source.

(d) The child may play the role of ally and support one or more family members, in their conflict with other members. Extreme examples are the child who feels compelled to stay up all night to protect mother from the alcoholic father when he comes home, or the child who is afraid to go to school lest the mother is physically attacked by the father. Children who are placed in the role of an ally and support to one family member, especially a parent, are likely to be in an anxiety-provoking situation in the first place. The anxiety is however compounded because their efforts will probably not be successful, since they seldom have the power and resources to provide complete protection.

2. There may be conflict between the family system's needs and the developmental needs of particular family members. Families require to develop and change over time. Following the creation of a family by the union of two people, the first changes occur with pregnancy and the birth of a child. From then on, whether additional children are born into the family or not, a continual process of change is necessary, as the family system as a whole adapts to the developing needs of the child or children. A family system that will meet the needs of a baby is different from that which will meet the needs of a toddler, a pre-school child, a primary school child, an adolescent and a young person ready to leave the family and perhaps start another nuclear family. Unfortunately family systems are not always found to be functioning in ways which facilitate, or even permit, the children in them to negotiate the various developmental stages successfully. The two main dangers are:

   (a) The system functions so as to infantilise the child, so that emotional development, and negotiation of the appropriate emotional milestones, are delayed.

   (b) Pressure may be brought to bear upon a child to shoulder responsibilities too great for the child's current age and level of emotional development. In these cases the child is forced into a pattern of prematurely 'grown-up' behaviour.

There are many family system patterns which may be associated with delayed emotional development of the family's children. A common one, as described in structural terms, is when there is an over-close relationship (called enmeshment by Minuchin[7]), between one parent and a child, and a relatively distant, or disengaged, relationship between the two parents. Most often the enmeshment is between mother and child and the father is found to be relatively uninvolved with the family, perhaps being a busy businessman who is seldom home. Enmeshment between one parent and a child can of course also occur when there is no other parent in the home. Under these circumstances the existing parent sometimes tries to make the child perform the role of the missing spouse which itself can be a heavy burden for a child and can give rise to anxiety. Circumstances such as these tend to delay children's emotional development. This can result in their being unable to cope with relationships and social functions of various sorts in age-appropriate ways. For example the child who has always been over-protected and babied by an anxious mother with whom he/she has been enmeshed may find it increasingly difficult to cope with rough children at school. This may lead to reluctance to go to school, with excessive anxiety associated with leaving home for school, so that ultimately a picture of severe school refusal may develop, as described elsewhere.[7]

It can also be anxiety-provoking for children to face pressure to grow up and shoulder responsibilities prematurely. This can happen in families where the parents are very much involved with each other, or with outside activities, and give their children insufficient affection, attention and support. Instead the children may be left to fend for themselves, both within the family and in coping with life outside it. This too can lead to anxiety which may however be repressed and expressed in other ways.

**Idiosyncratic Roles**

Various special roles for children have been described, but it may be that these are no more than descriptions of the way in which children come to act as result of the processes mentioned in sections 1 and 2 above. Labelling children's roles in this way has become less fashionable in recent years, perhaps because it tends to imply linear cause-and-effect relationships. Nevertheless some of the more commonly referred to of these roles will be briefly described.

The iodiosyncratic role about which most has been written is probably that of family *scapegoat*. This term seems to have been first used, in relation to family functioning, by Vogel and Bell.[8] It has biblical origins. In Chapter 16, verses 20–22, of the Book of Leviticus, Moses lays down how a scapegoat is to be used by the people of Israel. The priest was to lay his hands on the head of a goat and 'confess over it all their sins'.[9] After this had been done the goat was to be sent into the wilderness 'to carry all their iniquities upon itself into some barren waste'.[9] In fact the term has been used in family therapy in a way somewhat different from the process suggested by Moses. Thus the 'scapegoated' family member (often a child with symptoms), while appearing to be the person upon whom all the family's problems and difficulties are projected, is usually maintained in the family system rather than being sent out into anything equivalent to a barren waste. Some families depend on having a 'bad' child for their, often precarious, stability.

Another idiosyncratic role is that of 'parental' child. While it may be appropriate to give older children some parent-type functions in caring for younger children in the family, it is certainly possible to give too much responsibility to a child, as has been mentioned above. If this happens, and especially if the delegation of authority is not explicit, the child may become anxious and develop symptoms of various sorts. In extreme cases of 'parentification' there is reversal of roles, the child taking care of the parent, though the inversion of roles may be camouflaged.[10]

Other idiosyncratic roles which have been described include that of martyr, 'family angel',[11] sick member, handicapped member or 'disturbed' or 'crazy' member. Thus the martyr, through patient self-sacrifice, subjugates his/her interests for the good of the family. Gross[11] suggests that the 'family angel' performs a role analogous to that of the scapegoat, enabling family members to rally around in admiration, rather than condemnation. Nevertheless the role can be stressful since it is hard to be angelic all the time! The roles of sick, handicapped or 'crazy' family members are often associated with serious disorders of family functioning.

Minuchin and his colleagues[12] have described 'psychosomatic families'. These are families in which psychosomatic symptoms in one member, usually a child, comprise an important aspect of the way the family functions. In many cases there is already a 'primary' psychosomatic disorder, for example diabetes or a tendency to attacks of asthma, but these authors also describe 'secondary' disorders in which there is no evidence of a predisposing physical disorder. In either event the idea is that the role the child is playing is an anxiety-provoking one and the anxiety is expressed through psychosomatic symptoms.

The characteristics of 'psychosomatic families' are:

1. *Enmeshment*. In enmeshed families subsystem boundaries are weak and easily crossed, and individual members readily get lost in the system.
2. *Overprotectiveness*. In these families members have a high degree of concern for each others' welfare. They constantly supply nurturing and protective responses to one another and are over-sensitive to signs of distress in other family members. The overprotective attitude of parents can retard the development of autonomy, competence and outside interests in the children.
3. *Rigidity*. Minuchin and his colleagues use this term to describe the way these families endeavour to maintain the family *status quo*. Growth and change, as required for instance when a child enters adolescence, is difficult for them. Ways of interacting which are suitable for younger children cannot be abandoned in favour of those needed by adolescents. The need for change is denied and this tends to be associated with the appearance of symptoms.
4. *Lack of Conflict Resolution*. These families cannot resolve conflicts, partly because of their rigidity, which militates against change, and partly because of their overprotectiveness and sensitivity to each other's distress. Sometimes a strong ethical or religious code is the rationale used for avoiding conflict, but each family has its own way of avoiding facing up to conflict or of diffusing it without resolving it.

Minuchin and his colleagues[12] postulate that in psychosomatic families the child is in some way involved in a conflict between the parents; the parents may unite in concern about the child, thus avoiding conflict, or marital conflict is changed into parental conflict over the child, or the child may take sides or mediate. There is some independent support for the hypothesis of Minuchin and his colleagues. Loader and his colleagues[13] investigated family interaction in 12 families, each of which contained a child with eczema. They examined these families in relation to Minuchin's hypothesis, and also another hypothesis, put forward by various other writers, which they labelled the 'affective hypothesis'. They found that in 6 of the 12 families Minuchin's hypothesis was fully supported, and that it was partially supported in several others.

While studies of this sort present many methodological difficulties, it does seem that, at least in some instances, processes such as

Minuchin and his colleagues described can occur, and that psycho-somatic symptoms can be ways in which anxiety arising within the family system is expressed. It may well be that for this to happen there has to be a biological tendency, in the family member concerned, to develop the particular type of physical disorder involved.

## Attachment Theory and Anxiety in Children

Attachment theory is concerned with the making, nature and breaking of emotional bonds between people. Of particular importance in the present discussion is the nature of attachments that occur between family members, especially parents and their children. Bowlby[14,15] has investigated and described attachment phenomena. He holds attachment behaviour to be a biological phenomenon, characteristic of many primate species. Attachment theory conceives of the process of emotional bonding between parents and children, and between other humans, as being a class of behaviour at least as important as feeding and sexual behaviour, though it is distinct and different. It is because of attachment behaviour that families become systems, as described above. Emotional bonds may be likened to the glue holding a model together, except that they are usually much more fluid and flexible than glue which has set. Perhaps springs which can be stretched, distorted or even broken would be a better analogy. In the first year of life attachment behaviour is manifested by such behaviours as crying in the absence of the mother, calling, stranger anxiety and separation anxiety. All these behaviours tend to bring about proximity to the mother-figure.

Heard[16] has discussed the relationship between attachment theory or, as she calls it, 'the attachment dynamic' and family systems. She discusses the roles of 'care-giving' and 'care-seeking' behaviour which she considers in-built, interpersonal and complementary; and also exploratory behaviour which may be contrasted with attachment behaviour.

Exploratory behaviour becomes marked in the second year, once the child has started to walk, and is normally based upon a secure attachment to the person or persons (most often mother and other family members) to whom the child has become bonded.

In a normally developing child attachment behaviour is most marked during the second year, though it is important to know that it may be observed throughout life. Situations arousing attachment behaviour include those in which the individual is frightened or apprehensive beyond a certain degree; is hungry, tired, or experiencing physical discomfort; is unable to maintain access to and feels cut off from a home base and responsive, friendly people; or is faced with new or unpredictable experiences or change in familiar ones, to the extent that difficulty in handling the new situation is experienced. In these circumstances the care-giver assists the subject to deal with the situation and when there is a healthy outcome, the attachment behaviour lessens in intensity. With increasing experience of such situations the care-seeker's need to seek assistance progressively lessens, as does the frequency and intensity of the attachment behaviour. As this process proceeds exploratory behaviour then becomes increasingly possible.

Anxiety in children is liable to become marked and excessive when the care-giving by the person to whom the child is bonded is ineffective. Heard[16] describes two forms of ineffective care-giving: (a) care-giving experienced as underactive, fear-evoking and unresponsive; and (b) care-giving experienced as overactive, fear-evoking and impinging. Heard goes on to describe consequences of ineffective care-giving. The first of these is 'continuing unassuaged attachment behaviour'. If the care-giver is not able to provide the required form and type of care-giving, or if the interaction arouses the care-seeker's fears, for example if the care-giver becomes angry, attachment behaviour arousal may be intensified rather than diminished with, presumably, a continuing high level of anxiety in the care-seeker.

Heard also describes 'frustrated, inhibited and anxious exploratory behaviour', 'anxious exploration' and 'frustrated and inhibited exploration'. In all of these there is a failure of the care-giver to provide the care-seeker with responses necessary to terminate the attachment behaviour and relieve the anxiety which provoked it.

The use of attachment theory is but another way of looking at and attempting to understand some of the processes occurring in family systems. It can however sometimes be particularly helpful in understanding why particular children are anxious.

## The Child's Response

What determines whether a child in a stressful family setting becomes anxious, rather than depressed, behaviourally disturbed or psychotic? Constitutional factors in the child seem to play a part: some children are more anxiety-prone than others, while some may have a tendency to become depressed or to retreat into a psychotic world of their own. An anxious reaction in the child is also more likely if the general level of anxiety in the family is high. Yet another factor is the response which the child's reaction has upon the family system as a whole. Since we are dealing with circular processes rather than linear cause-and-effect relationships, this is a crucial issue. If the child's anxious state is part of a circular process by which the family's equilibrium is maintained, then it will tend to persist and perhaps increase.

Andrew was referred for psychiatric assessment because of extreme anxiety which appeared whenever he was due to go to school. For several weeks he had been unable to make it to school. The symptoms had worsened after his maternal grandmother, to whom his mother had always been very close, died quite suddenly. Father travelled away from home a lot and was seldom available to comfort his wife in her grief. This function therefore fell to Andrew. At interview he confessed that he was worried about what might befall his mother when he was at school; he even wondered if she might kill herself. Although Andrew's mother paid lip service to the desire to have Andrew attend school, in practice she readily acquiesced to his staying at home and indeed seemed glad to have him there. Andrew's anxiety about going to school thus had the indirect effect of enabling him to provide support and comfort to his bereaved mother. Only when the father was able to cease travelling away from home and to spend more time at home with his wife was it possible for Andrew to return to school. Once father was supporting mother, Andrew's role in doing so and the separation anxiety that enabled him to, were no longer required.

The manifestations of anxiety in children of families such as have been described in this chapter may take any of the forms described in Chapter 3. Thus the anxiety may be expressed overtly or it may be repressed and, through the operation of mental defence mechanisms, appear as phobic, obsessional, hysterical conversion of dissociative symptoms.

## The Implications of Family Dysfunction in the Assessment and Treatment of Anxiety in Children

Although the relationship between anxiety in children and

dysfunctional family patterns has only been sketchily outlined, it will be clear that the family system to which a child belongs is important in influencing the way the child's development proceeds, and whether or not the child develops acute or chronic anxiety of a pathological degree. A mental health professional who deals with an anxious child — or for that matter a child with any problems — and is not looking also at the family context is likely to be as successful as a gardener who ignores the type of soil, the amount of sunlight or the proximity of other plants when planting or attempting to nurture a flower. Assessment of the family system should therefore always be carried out in addition to interviewing child and parents. The interviewing and assessment of families is best learned through the observation of experienced family therapists, followed by supervised practice. A scheme for interviewing and assessing families is also set out in *Basic Family Therapy*.[4]

While there would probably be little disagreement among experts in the field on the desirability of *assessing* the family system, there might be less agreement on the matter of when *treatment* should address the whole family system, and when it should concentrate on the anxious child. There is a lack of data on which to base a scientifically valid answer to this question. Family therapy should, however, be considered when the following conditions apply.

(a) There are demonstrable problems in the way the family system functions. Determining whether this is the case is not always easy. It requires skill and experience in the assessment of families. The question becomes easier to answer, though, when the second criterion is also taken into account.

(b) The anxiety the child presents can be understood in the light of the way the family is functioning. Family dysfunction, however that may be defined, is not relevant in itself if its nature and severity do not appear to have a bearing on the signs and symptoms the child shows. But often the child's anxiety can be readily understood when the family system is assessed, as in the case of Andrew, mentioned above.

(c) The family is available and is willing to enter into therapy. It is not necessary to tell the family members that they are a 'disturbed' or in any way abnormal family. Such statements are seldom helpful, as well as being relatively meaningless, in that there is no valid definition of what is a 'normal' and what is a 'disturbed' family. All we can say is that certain families are organised in such a way that symptoms in particular members, for example anxiety in a child, are features of their current functioning. A more helpful approach is to say that the family, rather than being abnormal in some way or being responsible for the child's problems, can be part of the cure. This will often lead to the family's consenting to treatment.

It is not possible in this chapter to describe the various schools of family therapy, nor the family treatment methods available. Those lacking family therapy skills, in cases where a family approach seems to be indicated, should of course seek the help of experienced family therapists. Again, however, an outline of some family therapy treatment approaches is to be found in *Basic Family Therapy*,[4] together with references to sources of further information.

### Summary and Conclusions

The nature and way of functioning of the family system can be important in understanding anxiety in a child. Pathological degrees of anxiety in children are often associated with dysfunctional family situations. In such families children may be called upon to play stressful and idiosyncratic roles. These can lead to high levels of anxiety. When a family is functioning in such a way treatment of the child in isolation is likely to be insufficient to solve the problem. A look at family functioning, followed by treatment for the whole family group, is then often needed. Attachment theory is useful in understanding how family systems are formed and how the members relate together. If within the functioning of the family system, appropriate care-giving does not occur in response to children's care-seeking, while at the same time exploratory behaviour does not develop as it should, problems may arise in the development of the children's coping skills. These in turn may be associated with pathological anxiety. Family therapy may be the treatment of choice when the family system is such that the supports and care-giving are insufficient to enable the child to deal with environmental and developmental stresses without becoming unduly anxious.

## References

1. Von Bertalanffy, L., *General Systems Theory: Foundations, Development, Application* (Braziller, New York, 1968).
2. Hall, A. D. and Fagan, R. E., in *General Systems: Yearbook of the Society for the Advancement of General Systems Theory*, (L. von Bertalanffy and A. Rapoport, eds) (1956).
3. Beckett, J. A., 'General Systems Theory, Psychiatry and Psychotherapy', *International Journal of Group Psychotherapy*, **23** (1973), pp. 292–305.
4. Barker, P., *Basic Family Therapy* (Granada, St. Albans, 1981).
5. Barker, P., *Basic Child Psychiatry* 4th edn (Granada, St. Albans, 1983).
6. Epstein, N. B., Bishop, D. S. and Levin, S., 'The McMaster Model of Family Functioning', *Journal of Marriage and Family Counselling*, **4** (1978), pp. 19–31.
7. Minuchin, S., *Families and Family Therapy* (Harvard University Press, Cambridge, Mass., 1974).
8. Vogel, E. F. and Bell, N. W., 'The Emotionally Disturbed Child as the Family Scapegoat', in *A Modern Introduction to the Family*, N. W. Bell and E. Vogel (eds) (Free Press, Glencoe, 1960).
9. New English Bible (Oxford and Cambridge University Presses, 1970).
10. Skynner, A. C. R., *One Flesh: Separate Persons* (London, Constable, 1976), p. 417. (Published in USA as *Systems of Family and Marital Psychotherapy:* Brunner/Mazel, New York).
11. Gross, G., 'The Family Angel — the Scapegoat's Counterpart', *Family Therapy*, **6** (1979), pp. 133–6.
12. Minuchin, S., Rosman, B. L. and Baker, L., *Psychosomatic Families: Anorexia Nervosa in Context* (Harvard University Press, Cambridge, Mass., 1978).
13. Loader, P. J., Kinston, W. and Stratford, J., 'Is there a "Psychosomatogenic" Family?' *Journal of Family Therapy*, **2** (1980), pp. 311–26.
14. Bowlby, J., 'The Making and Breaking of Emotional Bonds', *British Journal of Psychiatry*, **130** (1970), pp. 201–10 and 421–31.
15. Bowlby, J., *The Making and Breaking of Affectional Bonds* (Tavistock, London, 1979).
16. Heard, D., 'Family Systems and the Attachment Dynamic', *Journal of Family Therapy*, **4** (1982), pp. 99–116.

# 7 ANXIETIES ABOUT DEATH: THEORY AND THERAPY

James W. Anderson

The impact upon children of news of a death confronts adults with a problem, since questions about death are not easy to tackle. Explanation of the phenomenon is impersonal and those who attempt it are aware that they have not answered the child's question. A description involves abstracting and objectifying, so an answer is bound to be as unsatisfying to the giver as incomprehensible to the receiver. When the question is limited to human beings, incompatible feelings around the same idea are aroused, for the death of some would be dreaded and that of others welcomed.

In psychotherapy practice, where we often deal with those who have been bereaved and with those who suffer a loss in the course of treatment, it is incumbent on us to talk informatively to the client about the effects of his experience. At times, he will convert by metaphor into phantasies about death current relationships with people which have lost their enjoyment or from which feeling has been dissociated. It is important to distinguish these two ideas, death as a symbol for loss of feeling about someone (including the client himself) and the actual death of a familiar person. Whenever investigators have tried to isolate the causes of adults' depressions, psychosomatic illnesses, depersonalisation syndromes and suicides, they have encountered the recurrent factor of a bereavement either in early childhood or in early adolescence just before the illness. Less is published in the way of treatment, but whatever the viewpoint of the therapist, it is nearly always advocated that the patient be re-confronted with the fact of the loss and his attitudes resulting from it. Careful use of words is called for, because death-imagery is freely used in psychoanalysis. Separations and prospective partings from loved ones and from the analyst can be reacted to as if they were permanent. Similarly, a boy's oedipal covetousness of his mother will be accompanied by hostile wishes against the father and dread of retaliation. An interpretation using death as a symbol may be the most vivid way of unbending the patient's message when the language of feeling comes hard to him or, as in the case of young children is simply not available. But if death in the practical sense is meant, the analyst is dealing with a different set of internal processes and therefore with imagery appropriate to different behaviour.

Nowadays, students of the effects of separation of mother and infant have quantities of excellent observations to draw upon. Since the publication of Bowlby's Monograph *Maternal Care and Mental Health*,[1] the fact that a separated child is one at risk both during the absence and for long periods afterwards has passed into common knowledge, giving rise to better techniques for handling unavoidable separations. The theory that has accrued is illuminating the normal infant's capacity for relationship with its mother, thereby benefiting the treatment of neurotic infants who have not been bereaved; it seems that behaviour characteristic of loss occurs irrespective of an actual separation from the mother.

Yet, our understanding of the infant's capacity to mourn will be blunted if his ability to comprehend the notion of death, which is a cognitive achievement, is not kept conceptually separate from it, a distinction which some clinicians ignore. Furman[2] for instance, considering the responses of young children to the mother's death as evidence for the possibility of mourning at young ages, argues that 'the understanding of death is a prerequisite to mourning' which implies that the experience of that form of suffering only attends the appreciation of its cause; and Brown,[3] struck by the high incidence of psychiatric maladjustment in persons following the death of a close relative, recommends a 'death-oriented analysis' in which the child's 'fear of death' might be discussed in therapeutic interviews in preference to an analysis aiming at sexual readjustment.

These arguments are unconvincing on several counts. First, they ignore the results of investigations into the child's discovery of death by psychologists such as Sylvia Anthony[4] who demonstrated that the death idea, a functioning entity with a form of its own, was not an explanation of responses to test items; it would be accurate to say that when a person's emotional development had reached a particular stage of complexity, certain aspects of external reality lead him to conceive of the idea and description of death; but not until seven to eight years of age did children understand the concept, apply it to human beings and elaborate it. Being dead is then part of the history of being a person. Her findings are in keeping with Piaget's views on the age and intellectual ability children must achieve before they are able to give an explanation of natural phenomena. Even so, there are people who throughout life appear to have accepted the finality of death but derive hope from the belief that the lost one will return or can somehow be reached. Nagy[5] showed that her sample of children believed that life and death could co-exist; after nine years of age they could accept that life ended in death, with the qualification that a soul might live on.

Second, it is a fallacy to say that mourning cannot be experienced until death is understood. There are three separate issues to be distinguished: (a) the subject matter of the child's experience; that is, the absence of the mother and the changes in the environment entailed by it; (b) the child's perception of the changed situation; and (c) his emotional state resulting from that perception. The prerequisite to mourning may well be the loss of the mother, but it is not her disappearing — which is an everyday event — that activates mourning: it is her continued failure to reappear. Motive and behavioural equipment to seek the mother are present and active, but the familiar figure on whom the child's responses to internal stimulation are consummated is absent. The *cause* of the processes in mourning is the child's appraisal of a situation in which his expectations are not met by the mother's return. The *experience* of mourning is a state of the organism which we customarily conceptualise in terms of feeling, such as distress, anger and despair; and *that which the experience is about* is the change in the external environment which an onlooker would specify in terms of the mother's whereabouts.

When the problem is set out in this way, speculation about the effects of a death can be replaced by descriptions of the child's behaviour at different levels in the causal chain. A study like Anthony's[4] deals with the validity of beliefs about death; she demonstrated that death acquires its emotional significance through its equation with separation. Although youngsters from three years onwards apply the word 'dead' to withered flowers, carcases hanging up and chopped insects, they are using learned associations, applying the verbal expressions of their parents to explain the changed appearances of living creatures when they have stopped moving. Soon sleep, the gaps in experience which sleep provides, the prone position and the inert generally come to symbolise death. Metaphorical uses proliferate, and a status hierarchy for whom or what death can be acknowledged begins with a simple sentiment like, 'It doesn't matter to kill worms', develops towards indifference to the fate of remote people, which contrasts with an attitude that denies the loss of high rankers through elaborate funeral ceremonies and religious beliefs asserting continuity. Death only becomes sorrowful when it symbolises the loss of the mother; fear of death is simply derivative of separation, or of the consequences of aggression and of talion punishment.

Information on processes of mourning will accumulate as we identify different moods from the behaviour exhibited by infants under stressful conditions, some of which are described below. Inspired by the example of Darwin's method of analysing emotional expression, ethologists now infer states of feeling from the pattern of behaviour in the natural circumstances in which it is shown. Since speech is a comparatively recent acquisition, our remote ancestors probably relied on social signals similar to those found in apes and monkeys; nonverbal signals like body posture, facial expression and movements towards and away from objects communicated relevant information when an emergency occurred; children would not have been understood unless their feelings had found outlet in signals which their guardians received as communications. However, even before the ethological revival had permeated child psychology, the disruptive effects of separating infants from their mother had been recognised, and observations of children undergoing the actual experience had begun to grow. The evolution of grief was seen to have three phases: one of furious protest when the child behaves as if the mother were likely to return; a second of despair when anger is masked by pathetic distress as if the futility of protest were at last realised; and a final stage of detachment, a listless turning away from the mother and indifference to her or any other human being's affection for him. Illustrated in J. Robertson's films, Bowlby's[1] account of the destruction of the infant's capacity for making an affectional bond organises the data we have about childhood loss, and Schaffer's[6] statistical record of infants' responses immediately after parting from the mother established the age of 28 weeks as that at which an attachment to the mother must be held to be established.

Material from psychotherapy sessions is relevant to the way in which feelings about a long-term relationship evolve in the transference to the therapist. Psychotherapy with children has convinced me that material with a destructive theme, and games with representations of dead people, are the consequence of an unexpressed anger, of their loneliness at being separated from a parent, or their feeling out of touch with their mother or father though no separation has in fact taken place. A child does not ruminate obsessively, as an adult might in the absence of an identifiable cause, on the prospect of perishing in illness or through other injury. For him, attacking, being attacked and feeling isolated underlie the anxiety overhanging the games in which dead objects feature. Indeed, I have noticed that children whose therapy-material uses the macabre are reluctant to replace those games with an acknowledgement of the conflicts that confront them in their everyday lives at home. As soon as those can be worked on in the transference, intense rivalries come to light.

Gerard, aged eleven years, was referred to me because of his unruly behaviour and poor concentration on schoolwork. His teacher was repelled by his pre-occupation with corpses, drawings of mutilated people, and his asking the teacher, whenever she left the room, if she were going to die. An adult feels reproached in the face of such odd communications. The effect of Gerard's strange play was to bring development of games with age-mates to a stop; so far from being an immobile child, he was hyperactive, yet his oddities had a paralysing effect on his interactions with friends. In psychotherapy, he put himself and the therapist alternately in the roles of killer and killed, jailer and jailed and would try to tie up or otherwise sadistically immobilise whatever opposed him. After some months of therapy, his perception of the situation between us no longer suggested to him that murder would take place; corpses disappeared from his paintings; instead, the obsene aspects of sex and scorn of the father's sexual and parental roles were repetitively flung at me, alternating with timid appeals for friendship or rescue. In school, the boy's learning achievements improved and although he remained a messy child and a bully to others, some feeling of gratitude was brought to life in his taking stock of his surroundings, in particular, the motives of people who cared for him. There was no notion of death, as an adult thinks about it, in Gerard's behaviour. The components of his attitude are those set out in Freud's account of substitutive formations in infantile phobias of animals. Little Hans refused to go out into the street because he was afraid of horses, but the material showed that what he was suffering from was not a vague fear of horses but a quite definite apprehension that a horse was going to bite him. In the replacement of his father by a horse, the child expressed his ambivalence to the man in a symptom which proved, by its consequences, to be socially alienating. If nothing were known about Little Hans's family background the formulation would end there.

The phobias of early childhood were a puzzle which Freud set out to disentangle in *Inhibitions, Symptoms and Anxiety*[7] a book which confronts the reader with two methods of approaching the problem. The first, Freud's question — 'What we want is to find something that will tell us what anxiety really is' — generated speculation on the nature of fear and anxiety which lasts to the present day. His second method, a biologist's one, was to state that all we could do was to 'examine the occasions on which infants in arms or somewhat older children show readiness to produce anxiety'. Manifestations of anxiety, he says, occur 'when a child is alone, or in the dark, or when it finds itself with an unknown person instead of one to whom it is most used — such as its mother'. These three instances could be reduced to that of missing someone who is loved and longed for. The danger situation which will evoke the signals of anxiety is the absence of the mother. When the infant finds out by experience that the presence of an external object, the mother, can put an end to the discomfort or the tension produced by growing internal stimulation, the danger it fears is displaced from that situation on to the condition which determined that situation, i.e. the loss of the object. A great step forward is made by the infant for his preservation, writes Freud, when anxiety appears in response to the absence of the mother, which is now the danger.

Unfortunately, Freud abandoned the naturalistic part of his theory in trying to elucidate the relation of anxiety to real danger on the one hand and to neurosis on the other. This dual commitment throughout the book prevents the emergence of a useful model. Realistic anxiety, he says, is anxiety about a known danger, i.e. one from an external object; neurotic anxiety is anxiety about an unknown danger, i.e. from an instinctual demand. Formulated in this way, the reader is left to speculate endlessly on what children are 'really' frightened of. Also, by classing fears as phobias, Freud's important distinction, that anxiety is a reaction to missing someone who is loved and longed for, was left for future writers to develop. For our present purpose — the possibility of death images persisting in young children's thoughts — it would be pertinent to expose some of the issues involved and to identify the sort of concept which might be useful.

## Children at Risk

The circumstances of the danger can be specified. Through damage to his body, the child could be rendered ineffective, unable ever to take part in the group's struggle for survival, and an impediment to its efforts. Or, with no discernible damage, he could fail to develop the social and communicative skills that bind the family, thus disrupting it by his demands, weakening its cohesiveness and mobility.

The natural environment provides dangers in the form of predators, fire and storms, events which are predictably a feature of the physical environment in which the child lives with his group. Other conditions of life include the amounts of food, heat and ventilation to which the group have become adapted; these amounts permit of a very small range of variations which, if exceeded, would constitute a threat to health or life.

When a child is separated from his mother, two broad areas of risk are created. One lies in these hazards of nature which he is exposed to when his explorations are unrestrained by the mother; in primitive society, when attack by animals is likely to have been the chief threat, a child would not have survived long at a distance from his mother or other care-taking person; the closer he would be to her, the more likely he would be to survive. In modern times, his vulnerability to damage by technological apparatus, illness and poisonous substances would be great without anticipatory, protective behaviour on her part. The second is the emotional effect on the infant of the loss of the mother, the attachment figure around whom his early learning is organised; a substitute might occupy her place but the abrupt change of environment could disarrange his developmental programme and prevent his co-operating with his care-taker. Although the ages at which separated children are critically sensitive to changes in handling remain to be accurately charted, it is beyond argument that their health and functioning may be jeopardised if they are separated from the adults who are caring for them during the years of their needing physical help from them. Hence, variations in the accessibility of the mother introduce two risk areas: the amount of protection available to the child, and the stability of his emotional development.

Many studies demonstrate that the frequency of neurotic and physical illnesses and of accidents to children correlate with the physical and emotional ill-health of the parents, especially the mother. From the day of the child's birth, he is liable to encounter withdrawn or overprotective behaviour of the mother's as part of her post-partum depressive reactions. A mother in that state has two major ways of perceiving and relating to the child; either he takes a specific but distorted meaning for her, whence develops a relation in which the child is viewed not as an individual in his own right, but as a being responding to the needs of the parent; or, without his having much specific meaning, the parent is so involved in her private concerns that she is unable to provide adequate mothering for the infant. Other workers have recorded that when a mother is absorbed in the misfortunes of her own relatives, her friends can be discarded and the family begin to withdraw from its social network; the father becomes impatient and uncomprehending or sometimes over-concerned, so that in addition to the anxious, episodic mothering that the child receives, non-complementary family roles are set up. The infant can be a competitor against the mother for care. Thus the sense of isolation produced by her unresponsiveness gives rise to anxiety that she will not be available when he needs her.

Similarly, the death of a member of the child's extended family, such as his maternal grandmother, though of little direct consequence to him, can affect his mother so profoundly that her responsiveness to him becomes permanently diminished. Then the occurrence of a death is not an isolated hazard to be coped with by disengaging or ignoring it, but a symbol of the change in the mother's feeling for him.

Broadening the focus reveals that a child's pathology cannot be understood only in terms of two-way relationships from child to parent. An event occuring to or an action performed by any member of the family may move the others so much that readjustment of functions will occur. If a family is split into subgroups, adaptability to changed circumstances prevents significant members from occupying their traditional roles. The approach from child to family pathology based on the disharmonious relationships and inappropriate functions performed by the separate members yields to the classification of styles of communicating that would formerly have been called delinquent, school phobic, or schizophrenic. The way in which a family functions to produce casualties has been conceptualised by R. D. Laing and others. The best-documented example is that of the schizophrenogenic family, in which the child is put into an untenable position by a mother whose injunctions elicit incompatible responses simultaneously and no other member intervenes to counteract her behaviour. In due course, the child develops the schizophrenic's inability to distinguish the logical status of his thoughts. It is of relevance here because of the fears and anxieties generated in children of intact families with apparently considerate parents.

To sum up; when we are uneasy about a child whose behaviour appears to be over-active or apathetic, or who is preoccupied with phantasy, and feel reproached or moved to help, it is likely that we shall have assigned him to a risk category which for convenience is formulated in emotional terms. The distinctions are important if distress is to meet with appropriate reactions. Seeing him hurry back to his mother in response to a loud noise or other unexpected disturbance that could result in body damage, we say that he is alarmed or frightened. If he shows distress at the absence of his mother and there is some obstacle preventing his regaining her, we describe him as anxious. When he is reluctant to approach and play with age-mates, we describe his state in vaguer terms like his 'being worried', 'in pain' or preoccupied and notice that he is unable to act without constant reference to his family, as if he were apprehensive at unspecified danger. Whatever the category of risk, scrutiny of the circumstances will reveal that the conditions giving rise to the infant's fear bear a close relation to those that are potentially harmful to him. (See Bowlby[9] for the basis of this theory.)

## Behaviour Indicative of Fear

As an example of the ethologist's manner of examining the occasions on which children manifest emotional behaviour, I begin with observations made on normal infants in their accustomed environments, taken from a study of attachment behaviour out of doors.[10] Although the aim of this study was to ascertain the distances that infants aged one to three years, when given unrestricted freedom, kept from their mothers, some instances of naturally produced fear were recorded. An infant of one or two years of age, when startled by a sudden loud noise or by an animal's behaving in an unpredictable way, would arrest his activity, fixate the stimulus, and back towards the mother, pressing himself against her, sometimes with his thumb in his mouth. When he is playing at a distance from his mother, say, at about one hundred feet, he will simply back away from the animal in any direction while fixating it, then walk or run back to his mother. But if the stimulus is a long way from him he stands still, points to the source of the disturbance, and looks towards his mother. These descriptions illustrate the distinctions which clarify the function of fear. The first is the role of the mother in generating the infant's response: she is a point in reference to which he re-positions himself. His attention alerted, he immediately turns his head towards her, aligning his body so that he can look alternately at her and the stimulus. Orienting himself to the mother has obvious advantages for his safety if physical help were needed from her, but it has an additional consequence which could colloquially be called giving courage: once he has taken a bearing on her and on the remote object, he is less likely to retreat; he will remain a while, appraising the situation, then perhaps set off to explore whatever it was that frightened him. If he is greatly alarmed, or is close to the mother when he gets frightened, he walks backwards or edges into her, focusing on the stimulus. Thus, when the child is frustrated, the mother has a role additional to that of reference point; the tactile contact which she permits provides him with a counteracting form of stimulation to terminate his distress. It may be significant that the mother displays very little concern in these mildly frightening situations. The behaviour sequence escape/retreat to mother/re-engage outside world results from the infant's own initiative.

I asked a control sample of volunteer mothers what frightened their infant and how he showed it. Their reports confirmed what was seen in the park: crying, turning to the mother, approaching and holding her is the typical response to alarm.

The commonest cause of distress mentioned by mothers of one- and two-year-old infants was the anticipated separation when the infant was about to be left with a friend of the mother's when she went out for a few hours. Although the infant was placed in friendly hands and said to be untroubled during his mother's absence, some mothers avoided hearing his protest by not telling him that they were going.

At one year of age, unexpected noises were frightening to three-quarters of the sample. By the time they reached two years, these infants had become habituated to most of the common sounds in their environment, but a specific noise such as that made by the sound of wind against a window pane, thunder, or trains going by could still evoke alarm. It seems as if sounds whose source cannot be located, and therefore oriented to, or cannot generally be predicted from appearances, remain perplexing to two year olds.

An infant's reaction to strangers is difficult to assess because it is not clear what degree of familiarity is implied in that relationship. Mothers use the term stranger to refer to any degree of acquaintanceship ranging from grandparents (who are living away) to passers-by, the criterion being the amount of time and recency of the period spent with the infant. Thus, the child's response cannot be judged without considering the stranger's subsequent behaviour, whatever the degree of kinship. Mothers say that their infant's withdrawal from strangers is no different from that of relatives whom he does not know. Even a father working away for a few days at a time can evoke fear when he returns home. Some children are selective in regard to strangers, recoiling only from those who have a loud voice, a wrinkled face, frizzled hair, or wear spectacles; some retreat from men but welcome women, and vice versa. Infants who approach strangers in the park may, when a stranger comes to their house, retreat to the mother. Infants who do not like strangers are capable of ignoring them if a playmate is present. Above all, there are fluctuations in the positive and negative reactions to strangers depending on the mood of the child, the moods having a link with his relationship with the mother; for instance, after a new baby has been born, an infant who shows no fear of strangers suddenly become cautious with them.

The well-known 'fear of strangers' concept over simplifies the position regarding infants' placed in novel situations. By the age of four months, nearly all babies will have discriminated their mother and shown reserve with other adults. Though many experiments demonstrate children's aversion from new people, I think that some of the withdrawal classed as fear of strangers is simply attention-seeking behaviour when the mother is in interaction with another adult in specific circumstances, such as his own home.

An extremely negative reaction can be produced by a familiar person to whom the child never became habituated, in spite of opportunities or, having come to like him, suddenly took an unaccountable dislike. A relative who called occasionally might evoke such a strong protest that he would stop visiting. It is characteristic of early life that once a percept is formed, it is localised in a setting and is extremely resistant to change, a process discussed by

Piaget;[11] in our example of the arrival of the semi-stranger, there is forced upon the infant's memory of a past perception the presentation of a significant stimulus which involves him in a forced 'recognition comparison'. Although the effects of this experience have not been documented for human beings, when animals are put into a situation where new input has to be matched against an incomplete model, the resulting tension can cause them to take flight.

Finally, a change in the appearance or behaviour of familiar things can evoke alarm behaviour. A mother who takes to wearing glasses evokes so much screaming that she leaves them off. A mother encountered in the novel setting of a hospital ward releases distress. Older children's imitations of bogey men or their using masks produces screaming until the disguise is discarded. The general principle is that a change in the appearance or behaviour of a familiar person which elicits a response incompatible with that elicited by the earlier version of the object causes in the child a state of uncertainty; there is a limit to the variations in the mother-image as to that of any other well-known object, that the child can tolerate without distress. Wolff[12] was unable to frighten his infants (aged up to six months) by wearing terror masks or by grimacing at them, but one mask of clear plastic that transmitted the colour and gross features of the face while obscuring any finer details, and a pair of spectacles that concealed the eyes, produced expressions of doubt and astonishment. Wolff concluded that a distortion of familiar facial configurations would provoke a fear response at that age.

It is clear that the possible outcomes of the state of being frightened are, at an early age, limited, but behaviourally they involve the immediate establishment of a closer relation with the mother. Any excessive stimulation, likely to be harmful to the organism, produced by unusual excitement of the receptors, or by the degree of complexity of the presentation, induces a state of alarm in the infant. Provided that the culture is one in which mothers tend to position themselves near their young, a population of infants who responded to alarming signals with a readiness to approach their mother would reduce their chances of injury in dangerous circumstances. As long as mothers do not leave the responsibility for maintaining proximity to the infant, as lower animals do in varying degrees, the outcome of infants' behaviour will have appropriate functional consequences. The closer he is to his mother, the mother to her group, and the group to its familiar territory, the greater the likelihood of his survival. My observations out of doors indicate that mothers, when not actually taking the initiative in remaining close, do position themselves in such a way that their infant's imperfectly developed ability to restore contact is facilitated.

In a study of fear, it is more informative to analyse those situations in which infants become alert, startled, timid and panic-stricken, and to look for the disposition of the mother, than to follow the old method of postulating specific phenomena like the darkness, animals or strangers and testing the belief that they take on a frightening significance during a phase of infancy. In middle childhood, the child is not frequently turning to the mother when he is alarmed and although the concepts of danger and of death are beginning to be understood, published studies of older children's fears do not list death amongst the objects evoking distress. Animals, the darkness, and storms are popular categories just after infancy, and then objects associated with parental warnings about accidents or story book accounts of wild animals persist.

**Distress**

While our infant at liberty is an exploratory, socially engaging creature, likely to confront any child or animal that catches his attention, if he is tired, in pain, or perplexed by the irreconcilable tendencies evoked in him by conflicting wishes, he withdraws interest from the outside world; his pace slows, he may become immobile or restless and his mother's nearness to him, so far from unleashing a challenging outlook makes only for further manifestations of attachment. The mother is the only provider of that kind of stimulation that can terminate his vacillations and reduce his discomfort; when he can reach her the time he spends beside her is longer than that when he is alert, and his unresponsiveness to the outside world finally merges with the state of sleep.

This pattern, which is phenomenally that of a child in a dejected mood, is an important one for our present purpose because of its affinity with the kind of distress seen in depression, the characteristics of which are different from those in adults. His indifference to surrounding attractions, whininess, bursts of restlessness, and lack of satisfaction from anything but the mother's caretaking is a close parallel, under natural conditions, to the behaviour seen in states of anxiety or apathy among children whose mother has been absent a long time or whose return to her is thwarted by their being kept away from home.

Ethologists identify states of feeling by specifying the situation which the child is likely to be appraising in the visible environment. Blurton-Jones'[13] book of ethological studies has many examples. Reddening of the face, for instance, is characteristic of a defeated child; a young child does not go red with rage. A blow delivered from the arm over face gesture by a frowning child occurs when, defeated, he cannot or will not escape. By interpreting such behaviour as a signal as to how another person's behaviour has been received, Brannigan and Humphreys[14] class signals not in terms of emotional causation but as an expression of the relationships between the parties which will follow the signal; our understanding of the form and content of such a signal is likely to be advanced more, say the authors, by stating that it has an 'appeasement function' than by postulating motives like fear or escape.

Andrew,[15] who studied mammalian signals from the point of view of the information the animal could potentially convey to another animal, observed that some expressions of dejection are derived from reflexes associated with immobility (the opposite of those preparing for exertion). The round shouldered hunch with limbs not fully extended, or crouched stance of the drowsy or depressed child is similar to the self-warming huddle in cold and tired mammals, just as in a dejected human being. As far as the mammal world is concerned, the adoption of a confident gait and stance with full limb extension is a sign of status. Andrew postulates reflexes, the functional converse of those predictive of exertion, which precede as well as accompany generalised motor inhibition. An example of immobility is freezing, which often begins with the animal crouched to leap and sometimes passes into more relaxed immobility; the development in forcibly constrained animals is comparable. Such inhibition, usually in a resting posture, also develops in an animal which is persecuted by a superior (when movements may be punished) or is tired or drowsy.

Other ethologists have noticed, from the pattern of movements in which the mood is embedded, that the most conspicuous unit is the change in the manner of locomotion; a dejected child does not go far from his mother and he does not run. He shows an absence of that focused attention which is a sign of confidence in social intercourse. Thumb sucking, ear-stroking, rocking and other self-comforting gestures engage the body and hands. No intention to do anything can be inferred from his actions, but the child behaves in such a way as to suggest to the onlooker that his condition has its causes outside the immediate environment.

Thus separate models are required to understand the causes and functions of distress. When it arises during fear, given in response to predators or other injuring agents, clues to its causes lie in the surroundings; the orientation of the child's body and sense organs indicate the source of the alarm, while the accessibility of the mother determines the outcome of the subsequent distress. But when we are referring to the distress manifested in states of dejection, anxiety or depression, we must use a model which takes account of circumstances beyond those which we can observe — of the 'off stage' phenomena as Leach[16] aptly calls them.

Whereas behaviour in fear is elicited by random events of short duration, evoking a response of relatively short duration (provided that the mother is accessible), anxiety and depression are lasting conditions occurring in response to a sequence of repeated events like frequent punishing, or over-rewarding, or prolonged failures of expectation like that caused by the loss of the mother, that is, by her continual failure to return.

The question is sometimes raised, at what point in time could a child during the separation period conceive of its becoming permanent in the event of his mother's dying, but I doubt if anything is to be gained by speculating along those lines; his decision would be the consequence of an intellectual appraisal made in retrospect when all possible facts, including his memories of the period, were available to him. When a child is bereaved of his mother, we have no reason to think that his protest at her departure, nor despair at the loss of hope in her rejoining him are at all affected by his trying to understand the nature of death. His reorientation to his surroundings depends on the capacity of the new attachment-figure to fulfil the functions of the mother; an explanation as to why the mother has gone away, or an indication as to where she is buried, is the information most likely to reduce searching and empty expectation.

The role of the care-taking adult is a peculiar one in that during the period of distress that attends the mother's departure, she is affronted by aggressive outbursts that she has done nothing to merit.

In field observations of mother-infant pairs, I found (although situations arousing the infant's anger rarely occurred owing to the trivial nature of such frustrations as his being prevented from playing at a forbidden place) that his being thwarted by his mother resulted in his maintaining a close proximity to her. Just out of arm's reach he glowers threateningly, strikes her and recoils, moves about restlessly in her vicinity and refuses physical contact when she tries to mollify him. Infants were never seen to be angry with anyone but the mother. They might snarl at an older child who interrupted their play, or occasionally push over an age-mate, but sustained rage was elicited by and directed only at the mother. The form of attachment behaviour seen when the infant is angry clearly has the purpose of coercing the mother to readjust her momentary goals and to reproach her for putting obstacles in his way. When she does not accede to his wishes or fails to amuse or distract him with another activity, his distress increases until signs of anger give way to expressions of despair.

To avoid their infant's prolonged distress, mothers usually adopt a compromise activity like feeding him or playing a game, which removes the persecutory aspect of being thwarted, whereupon secure attachment behaviour supervenes. Each party is motivated against prolonging the phase of angry attachment; from the infant's point of view, resumption of comforting tactile contact becomes possible, and from the mother's, the end of her being repeatedly confronted and hectored.

Interaction with the infant through a compromise activity may perhaps be learned slowly at first, particularly with a mother's first child, when her responsiveness to his initiative may not yet be tempered by her appreciating the advantage of ignoring some of his entreaties. As he ages, an infant's demands become more or less compatible with his mother's purposes, so that a relatively stable pattern of interaction develops to minimise the sorts of frustration that produce distress.

We do not have field data on the responses of infants to being thwarted by a substitute mother, but it is unlikely that the compromise activities she initiates, when confronted with an attack she has done nothing to elicit, do much to diminish the persecutory aspect of the child's frustration when he is still protesting against the loss of his own mother.

The term aggression, which is commonly used to imply destructiveness, calls for careful employment in case it should mask the function which angry behaviour, when oriented around a mother-figure, has in overcoming obstacles and in effecting those compromises which restore stable interaction.

In this and the preceding sections, I have described some features relevant to prolonged expressions of distress and suggested that if we separate the *cause* of the child's emotional behaviour from its *function* we are likely to clarify the disturbing situation, assign a category of risk, and alter those features of his environment which are producing stress. The interpretation of fantasy to account for young children's behaviour is, in my view, redundant until this prior analysis is carried out.

## Depression and Suicide

Examples of extreme distress appear in accounts of the fatally ill child in hospital, the impact of which on adults is so grievous and their inability to alter the course of events so demoralising that they are driven to postulate a sense of dying, understanding of which, they feel, would enable them to help to alleviate that form of suffering. 'In the more chronic dying experience, there is often evidence of depression, withdrawal, fearfulness and apprehension,' write Solnit and Green,[17] adding that future research in this area might examine how 'children express their knowledge or sense that they are dying' and to determine means of communicating with these children in a therapeutic manner. They quote the case of their terminally ill four-year-old patient Larry who had formed a trusting relationship with a young intern who cared for him during his repeated hospitalisations. 'On the day before Larry died, he asked the intern to hold him and said that he was afraid to die and that his doctor should come any time Larry needed him.' The astounded intern wondered 'how long Larry had known he was dying'. When the boy died twenty-four hours later in a coma, his parents reassured themselves by saying that Larry had not known he was dying. The intern thought that this was not true, 'but agreed that it was intolerable for the parents to realise that their only son had sensed his own approaching death'.

In their moving account of the child's deteriorating condition, the authors describe a number of circumstances, of which any one on its own would be sufficient to cause alarm and anxiety. Separated from his parents, confronted by unfamiliar figures in a strange milieu, he was subjected to unusual ways of feeding and of being handled. He was in pain from the illness, discomfort from the treatment, and expected bodily mutilation. He was immobilised, and frightened about what might be done to him under narcosis. When not drugged, he experienced boredom; his anger, roused by the separation, was neither dischargeable nor expressible in play. When his mother visited him, her greeting was modified by the state of quasimourning that she was in, as was that of the physician who attended him.

The authors say that Larry's greatest need 'was to be helped with a profound separation anxiety and depression' and this, of their conclusions, is in my view the correct one. The ways to approach this sad task, to modify the fearful fantasies that are generated by so much frustration might be fathomed, rather than postulate a sense of dying as an experience *sui generis*, with a special treatment.

Apparently convincing evidence of young persons' preoccupation with thoughts of death are contained in reports of the suicidal fantasies that sometimes accompany the mood of depression in adolescents. When feelings of hopelessness and inadequacy are connected with the belief that the child can do only bad things and that only bad things are expected of him, self-accusations and suicidal threats are expressed.

The fact that the suicide attempt is an act of self-injury which sometimes achieves self-destruction could plausibly support a hypothesis that the impulse to seek death or to fear and avoid death has instinctual force, this belief being deducible from early psychoanalytical writings. There are two conceptually distinct notions in metapsychological theorising. A classification of life and death instincts was evolved by Freud to support his clinical discoveries from which an impulse to *seek* death can be inferred. A *fear* of death postulated by Melanie Klein, derives from the experience of anxiety arising from awareness of aggression at an age when the distinction between self and outer world has not yet been achieved or when it has broken down. In either case, a conflict of forces within the organism, caused by a dread of dying, would constitute an argument supporting the connexion between the state of depression and suicidal behaviour, as if self-assault were the externalisation of advanced depression.

If the starting point for tracing this connexion is that feature in depression which appears as impoverishment of social contacts, there is apparent evidence that a continuum from socially isolated to suicidally inclined exists. Jan Tausch's[18] study of 41 suicidants aged 7 to 19 years in the early 1960s traces such a connexion. He estimates from his research among New Jersey Public School pupils that ten children make threats for each one who attempts the act and that nine serious attempts are made and fail for every one that succeeds. Although the act is aggressive, the individual is a lonely one who sees himself as inadequate to meet the demands of his society; or, if he is not withdrawn, he sees himself rejected by all about him and is unable to establish a close supportive relationship with any other individual. At school, he is capable of better work and in extra-curricular activities he takes little or no part. Jan Tausch did not think that children under nine years were pre-occupied with ideas of death. These children held a concept of life that extended after death and suicide was a means of saving face; alternatively, there might be an attempt to end pain from which no other resolution seemed possible. The difference between the attemptor who failed and the one who succeeded was the presence in the case of the one who failed of a person to whom he felt close. Added to the predisposing state of being depressed there were pre-cipitating events, minor psychosocial transitions occurring at the beginning and end of the school year: the pressures involved in returning to school after a holiday and the examination grade results were associated with the highest proportion of suicides.

The recovery phase of a mood swing as the most critical period for suicide is isolated by Faigel[19] whose report cites the fact that on college campuses, suicide is second only to accidents as a cause of death and twice as common as homicide as a cause of violent death in teenagers. He draws attention to the children's anger at parents or friends and their attempt to control and coerce those who would grieve at their death, the temper tantrums, disobedience, running away from home and truanting of those who contemplate death. Boys' use of firearms for self-destruction, their wrecking cars at high speed and other daredevil behaviour release great anger suddenly and violently, but this group have hysterical or socio-pathic personality disorders and are not profoundly depressed. There are warning signs beforehand in the shape of attempts at self-injury or accident-proneness.

To postulate depression to account for suicidal fantasies is mis-leading. It occurs when the word depression is used in different ways. Sometimes it refers to a mood, as when a person appears dejected, discouraged or sad; if he is chronically unhappy, he is said to be in a state of depression or to have a depressive illness. Diagnostically, the term is used to refer to a syndrome which includes a depressed mood, inhibition of action, unresponsiveness and liability to repetitive, self-reproachful thoughts. A state of depression is the commonest diagnosis made in respect of bereaved adults who present themselves for psychiatric treatment, but it is almost impossible to establish depressive illness before puberty owing to the children's marked mood swings; they may be extremely tormented, but are unlikely to reflect on the mood in the way that adults do. Used in a psychoanalytical sense, depression has its basis in the synthesis of destructive impulses and feelings of love towards the same object; obsessive self-accusations derive from the imagined complaints made by the injured love object.

One of the values of the surveys of suicidants is to lead our attention away from the ideation of introverted personalities, which is not necessarily predictive of future action, and direct it towards identifying character types from the population at risk. We gain a knowledge of the most important predisposing causes: broken homes, loss of a parent in early life and high illegitimacy rate; while in the case of intact families there is either a non-acceptance of the child or an imbalance in his upbringing resulting from mental illness in or social isolation of the family. The situations thus arising lead, in turn, to enduring mental states, the most common one isolated in the older literature being depression inferred from social withdrawal and in the later literature a 'hysteroid' disposition which develops into psychopathic behaviour. A parallel influence is that of the suicidogenous family, in which threats or attempts are part of a style of communication.

The most recent well-documented study is that by Otto[20] in which a 1955–9 sample was followed up until 1969. Otto collected information on 1727 suicidal attempts by Swedish youngsters aged under 21 years. His analysis suggests that the suicidal act has the character of a punishment or is intended as a threat against people in the environment, aiming at provoking guilt in closely related persons. Through his attempt, the suicidant makes a call for help, an appeal for engagement, and the environment reacts in the expected manner. The prominence of passive methods with a relatively slight risk of a fatal issue is another indication that the suicidal attempt is aimed at impressing the environment rather than actually causing death. Depression was not a common diagnosis; 'infantile' and 'hysteroid' personalities predominated as diagnostic categories, that is, people characterised by immaturity, impulsiveness, egocentricity and at the same time by role-playing, dramatising behaviour. The self-destructive message was delivered particularly when a psychosocial transition occurred. There was an increased frequency of suicide in children towards the end of the summer vacation just before the beginning of the new school year, and amongst conscript adolsecents towards the end of their furlough when faced with a return to their unit. Young conscripts had made frequent visits to the Medical Officer, school children to the school nurse. Compared with a non-suicidal control group, child and adolescent suicidants of both sexes had considerably more entries in the Register of asocial behaviour kept by the Penal Authorities. Attempted suicides had also a higher sick-listing frequency for both mental and physical causes as recorded by the social insurance scheme. It was possible to earmark a group at special risk in respect of renewed attempts and other developmental casualties by consulting the recorded sick-listing frequency, which was particularly high for boys and girls aged ten to thirteen years, with boys higher than girls; this also applied to children and adolescents for whom no plausible explanation of external events was recorded but for whom the act was attributed to a condition of mental illness. For those who had made suicidal attempts because of school problems, during military service or in connection with pregnancy, the sick-listing frequency was negligible.

It is encouraging to learn from Otto[20] and from other researchers experienced with this type of crisis, that a treatment plan does not call for deep knowledge of the individual's motives and that in most cases a profound psychotherapy is unnecessary. The suicide attempt is often impulsive. By admitting the child to hospital, we remove him from the social situation that forms the background to his attempt and can then spend time in dealing with the parental inter-relationships. Even in a state of mourning, there are ways of adapting to loss which are facilitated by an environmental manipulation providing support during the crisis period. It is only when a pattern of disorganisation cannot be identified that there is justification for prolonged analysis of the individual.

## Conclusions

The fact that most children persevere in behaviour that results in their survival is not a reason for thinking that they dread death. When at a fact-finding stage, curious about the world around him, the child may ask questions about it and curiosity will be heightened by the death of someone he is fond of. But if he shows a preoccupation with his or someone else's dying, there are different levels of investigation open to us. We can try to see what situation he is appraising, in particular, the disposition of his mother, her accessibility, her state of health and her relationships with her support-figures, such as her spouse and relatives. There are different trains of consequences if a brother or sister dies. The gist of the published studies is that the child's response is formed largely from the cues given in the reactions of the adults around him rather than from his own feelings about the loss. Sometimes he is caught up in the implications of other misfortunes to his kin, such as unemployment or mental illness, occurring in a family which is unable to use its resources for recovery. If he persists in ruminating about death, the ethological model is useful to assign a category to his associated behaviour by embedding it in a social context; this suggests environmental alterations, which is in keeping with the general thesis that morbid fantasies are helpfully explored in relation to current stressful events, especially those taking place within the family.

## References

1. Bowlby, J., *Maternal Care and Mental Health* (WHO, Geneva, 1951).
2. Furman, R. A., 'Death and the Young Child', *Psychoanalysis*, Study of the Child XIX (1964).
3. Brown, F., 'Bereavement' in A. Gould (ed.), *The Prevention of Damaging Stress* (Churchill, London, 1968).
4. Anthony, S., *The Child's Discovery of Death* (Kegan Paul, London, 1950).
5. Nagy, M. H., *The Meaning of Death*, (McGraw Hill, New York, 1965).
6. Schaffer, H. R., 'Objective Observations of Personality Development in Early Infancy', *British Journal of Medical Psychology*, 31 (1958), pp. 178-83.
7. Freud, S., *Inhibitions, Symptoms and Anxiety* (Revised edn) (Hogarth Press, London, 1926).
8. Benedek, T., 'Towards the Biology of the Depressive Constellation', *Journal of the American Psychoanalysis Association*, 4 (1956), p. 389.
9. Bowlby, J., 'Reasonable Fear and Natural Fear', *International Journal of Psychiatry*, 9 (1971), pp. 79–88.
10. Anderson, J. W., 'An Empirical Study of the Psychological Attachment of Infants to their Mothers'. Thesis presented for the degree of Ph.D., University of London (1971).
11. Piaget, J., *The Construction of Reality in the Child*. (Basic Books, New York, 1937, English translation 1954).

12. Wolff, P. H., 'The Natural History of Crying and Other Vocatizations in Infancy' in B. M. Foss (ed.), *Derterminants of Infant Behaviour* vol. IV (Methuen, London, 1969).

13. Blurton-Jones, N., *Ethological Studies of Child Behaviour* (Cambridge University Press, Cambridge, 1972).

14. Brannigan, C. R. and Humphries, D. A., 'Human Non-verbal Behaviour, a Means of Communication' in N. Blurton-Jones (ed.), *Ethological Studies of Child Behaviour* (Cambridge University Press, Cambridge, 1972).

15. Andrew, R. J., 'The Information Potentially Available in Mammal Displays' in A. A. Hinde (ed.), *Non-verbal Communication* (Cambridge University Press, Cambridge, 1972).

16. Leach, E., 'The Influence of Cultural Context on Non-verbal Communication in Man', in R. A. Hinde (ed.), *Non-verbal Communication* (Cambridge University Press, Cambridge, 1972).

17. Solnit, A. J. and Green, M., 'The Child's Reaction to the Fear of Dying', in A. J. Solnit and S. A. Provence, (eds), *Modern Perspectives in Child Development* (International Universities Press, New York, 1963).

18. Jan Tausch, J., *Suicide of Children 1960–63* (New Jersey Department of Education, undated).

19. Faigel, H. C., 'Suicide Among Young Persons', *Clinical Pediatrics*, 5(3) (1966), pp. 187–90.

20. Otto, U., 'Suicidal Behaviour in Childhood and Adolescence', in J. Waldenstrom *et al.* (eds), *Suicide and Attempted Suicide* (Skandia International Symposium, Stockholm, 1972).

## Further Reading

Hollingsworth, C. E. and Pasnau, R. O., *The Family in Mourning* (Grune & Stratton, London, 1977).
Torrie, A., *When Children Grieve* (Cruse Publication, 1978).
Toynbee, A. and Koestler, A., *Life After Death* (Weidenfeld and Nicholson, 1976).

# 8 SPIRITUAL ANXIETY AND ITS CURE IN CHILDREN

Eamonn F. O'Doherty

To understand 'spiritual anxiety', it is important in the first instance to distinguish between guilt feelings on the one hand, and true guilt on the other. The infant and the child can and do experience guilt feelings, but true guilt does not exist until late childhood. Moreover, guilt feelings are of different kinds and intensities. It will be remembered in this context that Freud distinguished three different kinds of anxiety: reality anxiety, which arises because of real dangers of the external world; neurotic anxiety, which is the fear of internal dangers, particularly the fear that the ego will be overwhelmed by the demands of the instincts; and moral anxiety, which is related to moral conscience proper. These three categories of anxiety relate also to different categories of guilt. Real guilt is the existential status of the person in respect of behaviour carried out *sciens volens* which is intrinsically wrong. Real guilt exists in direct proportion to one's standing as a person. The more mature, the more intelligent, the more free, the more culturally endowed, the greater will be the level of real guilt. Conversely therefore, the infant and young child will not incur real guilt, by reason of immaturity, undeveloped intelligence, rudimentary freedom, and lack of formation.

## Emotional Guilt

Emotional guilt, the guilt feelings referred to above, admits of many degrees, and in childhood is rarely morbid. It is a complex mixture of many different emotions and feelings: a sense of rejection, a dread of and desire for expiation and reacceptance, fear, self-reproach and many others. Even when the child uses apparent moral categories of good, bad, right, wrong, it is important to remember that he is using these words in child's concepts meaning acceptance, rejection, reward, punishment, affection given, affection witheld. These categories are functions of the pre-moral

128

conscience as distinct from the superego. The distinction is this: superego functions exclusively on the plane of emotions and is largely unconscious, while the premoral conscience is simultaneously a conscious cognitive evaluation and an evaluation in terms of conscious felt states of emotion.

Emotional guilt is not in itself a morbid state. It is a normal experience of the developing child. However, it can become neurotic in two ways: the first is when the guilt feelings reach an intolerable level of anxiety. The second is when guilt feelings are experienced in an obsessional way. Both these phenomena are found in relation to what we shall call spiritual anxiety in children.

## The Primordial Fears

Ever since Kirkegaard, Karen Horney, and the spread of existentialism, it has become a commonplace to acknowledge that anxiety is intrinsic to the human psyche. *L'angoisse c'est la vie*. There is not just one anxiety however. One can distinguish several different kinds of primordial anxieties even in childhood. On the whole one can say that these primordial anxieties spring from the experience of one's finiteness and dependency and from the bewildering unknown present and future. The infant and child are not afraid *of* the dark but of the unknown danger that may be lurking in it. We shall call this anxiety the fear of the unknown. The second of these primordial or universal anxieties is related to Freud's neurotic anxiety above, although it is not in itself neurotic. It is due to the experience of one's own emotions, and particularly in childhood, one's inability both to understand and to control them. One has only to observe a three year old in a tantrum to understand this point. This anxiety we shall call fear of instinctual life. The third of these primordial anxieties is the fear of death. Recent literature has shown that death and the fear of death play a much greater part in the child's world than was reckoned with even a generation ago. Margaret Mead pointed out some years ago that a whole generation of children in the fifties and sixties had grown up in USA without ever having seen or heard anything connected with death. In her memorable phrase (personal communication): 'For too long children have been given the facts of life. It is time they were given the facts of death'. Because they were not given the 'facts of death', Margaret Mead pointed out that they created their own frightening fantasies of death. It will therefore readily be seen that these three fears, the unknown, instinctual life and death lie at the heart of the experience we call spiritual anxiety.

## Fantasy, Magical Thinking and Religious Belief

Two of the most difficult problems the child has to solve are the relation between self and acts and between self and the real world. Both these problems are solved by the gradual discovery by the child of *ego* as initiator of behaviour and as the referral point of experience, but this discovery requires a long protracted voyage of discovery. The two best-known stages on the way are the discovery of the difference between fantasy and reality on the one hand, and the discovery of the limitations of finiteness on the other. The first of these is best illustrated by the survival of the Santa Claus myth up to the middle childhood in spite of all the reality evidence and the pain of relinquishing the fantasy. The second is best illustrated perhaps by the acceptance of the Cinderella myth, 'the fairy god-mother', who can do anything and the survival of this myth into the adulthood even of many scientists illustrated by the Uri Geller mythology of spoon-bending by psychic means. The relevance of this to spiritual anxiety lies in the very great difficulty on the adult's part to decide at what point and in what way religious doctrines of the supernatural are distinguished by the child from Jack and the Beanstalk or from his own dreams, and to what extent the child can distinguish between the magic of fairy tale and the power of God in the scriptures. The danger in terms of spiritual anxiety is twofold: on the one hand, a failure to make these distinctions can leave the child haunted by demons, witches, and things that go bump in the night, in other words, the assimilation of supernatural realities into fairy lands forlorn. The second danger is that the child may assimilate the doctrines of religion into his own literal thinking, and in this way make these doctrines part of his own finite empirical world, thus precipitating fears that he cannot cope with.

## The Nature of Spiritual Anxiety

In the strictest sense there is no such thing as 'spiritual' anxiety but rather anxiety centring around a spiritual focus. The anxiety itself is not different, except perhaps in its intensity, from any other anxiety. It is most likely to arise between the end of latency and the onset of puberty, and again at mid-adolescence, but this latter age-range is outside the scope of this article. During latency it is unlikely to arise simply because the child's emotions are dormant and his attention is focused on the external world. Between seven and ten, the child is very likely, in Western cultures, to be given for the first time perhaps, the vocabulary of religious doctrines concerning God, creation, Heaven, Hell, life after death, a sacramental system and the great archetypal stories from scripture. Teachers, preachers and ministers of religion are on the whole better equipped now than in former generations to distinguish between their own conceptual understanding of the words they use and the possible erroneous interpretation of the same vocabulary on the part of the receptive child. One can illustrate this, not perhaps from the contemporary scene, but from some historical examples. Puritanical movements in Christianity exaggerating the notion of sin and extending it beyond reasonable theological limits are one example. Fundamentalist interpretations of every comma and word of the bible in a purely literal sense are another. Conflicts between Ayatollah Khomeini's Islam and the She'ite Muslims are another. One perhaps can include here the Hindu doctrine of Krishna and his many instantiations as seen by a Hindu child on the one hand and an adult Brahmin on the other.

## Sin in the Child's World

On the whole the child seems to think that there are only two sins: disobedience and telling lies. All other misdemeanours can be subsumed under these two concepts. It should be pointed out however that the child's use of these words can mislead the adult world. Many a priest has heard a child say 'I was disobedient five times, and I didn't do what my mother told me'. It is also important to remember that the child's understanding of 'telling a lie' is not at all that of the adult. One has frequently observed a child answering 'No!' with great vehemence when asked 'Did you do this, that or the other?' and then breathe quietly 'Yes' to himself to cancel out the 'No'. Spiritual anxiety however can arise and indeed does arise when a child fails to operate this form of childish magic and experiences instead intense guilt feelings with which he cannot cope. The child cannot distinguish different degrees of magnitude of wrongdoing except in a childish way. Thus, to break a trayful of glasses accidentally and with no responsibility whatever attached to it is a much greater sin than to break one glass deliberately. In the same way the more fantastic the content of a lie, the greater the guilt of lying. It seems clear therefore that to attach the concept of sin and punishment for sin to the child's thinking in these matters may precipitate very severe spiritual anxiety and lead on to 'scruples'. On the other hand, as in the case of James Joyce and the hellfire sermon in *Portrait of the Artist as a Young Man*, inability to cope with the intensity of the anxiety precipitated can lead to the abandonment of all religious belief.

## Scruples

The word 'scruples' is used in two very different meanings just as the word 'guilt' is. On the one hand scruples in the theological sense is a spiritual trial, an agony of doubt and uncertainty about sin and real guilt, and involves an obsessive concern with observing the minutiae of 'the law'. In this sense sometimes gifted and holy persons seeking perfection may become scrupulous without any suggestion of mental illness. The second usage of the word however is relevant here. In this second usage 'scruples' refers to obsessional thinking and compulsive or near-compulsive behaviour as a means of coping with spiritual anxiety. Several examples come to mind: the child who refuses any food or drink which appears to her to have a black spot in it or on it (cf. Lady Macbeth 'Out, out dark spot') is trying to come to terms with the imagery of sin as a stain on the pure whiteness of one's soul; the child who repeats a simple prayer formula over and over again until he gets it just right to his own satisfaction is confusing prayer with magic ritual and may be trying to expiate the guilt feelings attached to some imagined violation of taboo. Depending on the intensity of the anxieties precipitated in the child's mind in these ways, emotional scars may be left for the rest of the individual's life.

## Taboo and Ritual

In the sphere of moral behaviour, many adults even in contemporary cultures, still think in terms of violation of taboo and ritual expiation. How much more therefore will this be true of the child's thinking. A taboo is a prohibition which depends for its enforcement on the precipitation of intense guilt feelings and the desire for punishment, even when there is manifestly no moral responsibility present. Freud used this concept in describing the oedipal phase of the child's development. Violation of the taboo is so dreadful that no reason need be given for the taboo itself or for the punishment that follows its violation. We can see at once how the concepts of sin, wrongdoing, responsibility, and punishment, even by a loving God, can be interpreted by the child (and by many contemporary adults) in terms of taboo rather than in terms of reasonable responsibility consciously incurred for behaviour cognitively understood to be intrinsically wrong. Thus punitive toilet training can lead to excessive guilt feelings and spiritual anxiety in the sexual sphere between latency and puberty, and indeed may last into adulthood. Ritual, in the technical sense, is standardised, repetitive, overt behaviour, by means of which the individual seeks to evade or to reverse the consequences of violation of taboo. One can see this clearly in the behaviour of a child who may create his own magic ritual to restore the equilibrium lost through the violation of the taboo. This sequence can easily be misinterpreted by the adult world as repentance, confession and expiation. The child who is punished for striking his sister and then is forced to say to her 'I'm sorry' before being readmitted to the family circle, may perceive this sequence of events precisely as the violation of a taboo and a magic ritual of forgiveness.

## Cure

Spiritual anxiety, as we have been dealing with it so far, is not itself an illness (although it may lead to illness later on), and therefore the word 'cure' may be inappropriate. Clarification, reassurance, and supportive love are the appropriate concepts. Clarification: this demands two processes on the part of the adult, be he therapist, teacher, parent or minister of religion. The first is the necessity of trying to understand what the words and concepts so clear to the adult may mean in the child's mind. The second process is the necessity of de-emotionalising the essential doctrines of religion. This applies equally to all the great religions.

De-emotionalising, meaning the elimination of or at best minimal-ising the emotional charge of religious imagery is closely related to, but is not identical with, the concept of de-mythologising.

Reassurance: there seems to be no doubt that the precipitation of emotional guilt feelings and of spiritual anxiety in the sense defined was used in the past and presumably is still used today as a control mechanism to regulate the behaviour of children, much as the ghosts of the ancestors sitting perpetually in the rafters were and are used as a control mechanism over the children of the Manus. The use of religious teachings in this way is an unhealthy misuse of what ought to be sublime doctrine taught for its truth value and not for its control value. Reassurance means the process whereby the child's fears, ghostly imagery, bewilderment in the face of the incomprehensible, are allayed by the strength and clarity of the adult's religious stance. In this context, perhaps the most important contribution psychology can make is the elimination of the possibility of experiencing the non-experienceable: disembodied spirits, angels, devils, God himself, flying saucers, little green men and extrasensory perception. It is sometimes thought that concepts of spirits etc., are intrinsic to a supernatural faith. There is a sense in which this is true: the sense in which the concept of spirit is the concept of the possibility of a wholly non-material being outside the space-time continuum and independent of it, and therefore outside the possibility of being experienced sensorially. However, this is not what it means to many adults, (psychic researchers, spiritualists, some charismatics, etc.). The child's intellect is incapable of conceiving spirit in the former way and therefore assimilates it to fairies, hobgoblins, science fiction and other fantasies. Reassurance means having the determination, the honesty and the clarity to make clear to the child the fictions involved in such fantasies and to distinguish these completely from the contents of religious belief.

Supportive Love: in the Judaeo-Christian tradition, as indeed in Greco-Roman mythology, the image of a punitive God has some-times predominated over the Good Shepherd, loving father image. The expulsion from paradise, 'vengeance is mine' saith the Lord, hellfire for all eternity, and the presence of uncomprehended evil in the world, are all part of the punitive God image. It is true that some preachers in the past and present, may have used such imagery to precipitate spiritual anxiety in their followers. What is more true however is a distortion in the other direction, the precipitating of guilt feelings, self-reproach, intense spiritual anxiety, by the use of mass meeting stimuli in the hands of gifted evangelisers, to produce sudden and short-lived conversions whereby the guilt-feelings could be expiated by public confession and abasement. Supportive love knows none of these things. Essentially is is the process whereby God's love for man is mediated through the significant adults in the child's world to eliminate spiritual anxiety.

# 9 UNDERSTANDING AND COPING WITH ANXIETIES ABOUT LEARNING AND SCHOOL

Elsie L. Osborne

The aim of this chapter is to look at anxieties which arise from the nature of the school situation itself rather than at anxious children in school. Where examples of individual children are given they are not necessarily intended to be typical of most children but rather, to illustrate through them the kind of problems which children face in the course of normal school life. The fact that most of them find their own resolution to such problems is commonplace of course. However, the study of cases where help was needed does seem to have implications for the way in which the schools themselves might attempt to recognise and manage some of the more identifiable risks.

The recognition of the unspoken anxiety of young children in hospital led to change in priorities, and indeed, improved the rate of recovery.[1] By concentrating on better preparation, on the provision of a familiar figure to support the child, and the readier acknowledgement of unhappiness in the ward, immense changes have been achieved. It is suggested that these findings might also have relevance for education.

The work of Bowlby has undoubtedly been more important than any other in drawing attention to the importance of the young child's first separations from mother.[2] In the debate about this, less attention has been paid to the relevance of attachment theory for learning. However, Ainsworth[3] has developed the theory's implications, in this respect, pointing out the greater readiness of the child to explore, to discover for itself, and therefore to learn, when it has a secure base to which it can return at any time. The author's own observation reinforces Bowlby's notion of an 'invisible elastic band' between the child and its mother.

Many studies are concerned with children's behaviour in response to various situations. One of the additional contributions of attachment theory is the possibility it provides to understand the anxiety associated with such situations, by linking the study of intrapsychic development with the context within which that

136

development takes place. It is especially relevant to the progress towards autonomy which is the aim of education.

## Starting School

The work of Bowlby and of the Robertsons is particularly important in relation to the first of the major transitions most children experience, that of starting school.

It is not surprising that with or without theoretical backing, most nursery and infant schols have attempted to take special account of these transitional aspects. The author's own experience suggests that many teachers are very well in touch with the need for sensitive management of first entry into school. The need for a familiar adult as a continuous figure has been implicit in the organisation of the primary school, with one teacher to one class throughout the year.

For most children now the first experience is more likely to be into nursery or play group at three or four years rather than at the age of five years, when compulsory schooling begins.

A study of this first, pre-school, transition[4] quotes a figure as high as 74 per cent of children in some form of pre-school group by the age of four years. Provision is, of course, of many kinds and more or less satisfactory, with parental preference only partially met.

Their survey gives an account of the strategies nursery staff adopted in order to ease school entry. These included staggered entry, having mothers stay whilst their children settled as well as visits to the nursery beforehand. Apart from this, plans for helping children to adjust were not usually thought through in advance, and contacts between parents and staff were in many ways unsatisfactory. The lack of meaningful involvement of parents is seen as starting a process of separation of the two worlds of home and school which continues to grow subsequently.

An interesting finding was that children whose mothers spent most time in playing with them at home, engaged in more interaction with other children and in more imaginative, dramatic play when they entered school. The authors felt their results supported the view that 'a more intense relationship with their mothers is likely to be reflected in a general social orientation towards other children,' and that security of attachment between child and mother correlated with social competence with their peers.

It is worth noting that this result comes from an empirical study, with cautious conclusions, and with a starting point well removed from attachment theory.

A more informal and personal study, much more influenced by the Robertsons' work on transition into hospital is provided in Janis.[5] In this the family friend of a two-year-old observed this little girl's entry into nursery school, and her subsequent adjustment over the following year. It shows how, even for a child without major problems, the separation from mother was often painful, and it gives a vivid and sensitive picture of a little girl's anxieties.

One further example underlines the importance of a single familiar adult to a child's capacity to learn. This time the context is a very different one. In contrast to the nursery schools and play groups for normal children described in the previous references Holmes[6] addresses herself to one of the most deprived groups of children in our society.

In an article on the effectiveness of educational intervention for pre-school children Holmes describes a special unit for 3-year-olds in day and residential care. The unit involved the children in daily attendance for 1 to $1\frac{1}{2}$ hours in small groups of four or less, with a qualified nursery teacher, preceded by several weeks of a daily half hour for each child alone. The children were chosen by the staff because they were already showing difficulties in learning as well as behaviour. The teacher took particular care to listen and respond to each child individually and to allow no comments to go unheeded.

The results for this very deprived and vulnerable group are significant for the understanding of the ordinary development of young children also. At school entry the special group had significantly increased their language development, their ability as measured by intelligence tests, and a year later none had been singled out by their teachers as presenting a problem. This compared with a control group whose failure to adjust to ordinary school was accompanied by serious learning and behaviour difficulties.

Translated into the management of the more ordinary anxieties of children starting school it would seem likely that here also the teachers' efforts to form an ongoing and attentive relationship are crucial.

## The Entry into Primary School

Even when there has been good pre-school experience the entry into infant school requires further adjustment, with fresh anxieties. In a companion DES/NFER research study to Blatchford *et al.*,[4] the discontinuities between the two stages, pre-school and primary school were highlighted.[7] The importance of various features in order to ensure continuity were identified, including the aims of the staff (e.g. the blurred distinction between care and education); the provision of materials, the segmentation of the daily programme, the jump in the range of activities and where the emphasis lies and the children's degree of choice.

Problems could arise not only for children unfamiliar with the new demands of activities centred on literacy and numeracy but also for those who had experience which meant they were already too familiar with, for example, the school's initial reading scheme.

Strategies are suggested for easing these discontinuities but the authors point out that these are permeated and transcended by personal relationships. The recommendations for dealing with this aspect of the transition are very close in spirit to the issues already raised in this chapter. The need for the child to feel expected, to have his own peg and drawer, to be recognised and named by his teacher, reassuring him and offering frequent short bursts of attention, explaining unfamiliar sights and events, introducing him to other adults he will meet and dealing with absences and other critical events with extra sensitivity.

Familiarity, continuity, feeling known and expected are the constant themes associated with reducing anxiety for the normal child.

The special problems of the deprived child, however, need special solutions and a development of a particular ILEA (Inner London Education Authority) based project is contained in Boxall.[8] The Nurture group approach is now well known and has long since moved from experiment to established practice. The deprived group with which it is concerned are described as those children who have not had normal relationships in early childhood and are emotionally and socially younger than their age. Many have severe personality and behavioural problems, disturbing and anti-social. The educational nature of the approach is strongly emphasised by the psychologist who developed it, the skills used are those of teachers and the programme takes place in normal schools.

The work is based on the attachment of the child to the teacher in a much more dependent way than would normally be contemplated even in the most accepting infant reception class. The establishment of trust and an atmosphere of safety allows for the growth of demands from the teacher, who from secure dependency can develop independence and learning. To quote Boxall:[8]

> Anxiety is thus reduced, and teacher and helper are enabled to draw maximally on their own resources and are not inhibited by feeling that somewhere there are experts who know better. . . . The work is approached with confidence and they (the teachers) grow with the children. The relief to the other teachers is considerable and a greater sense of community develops in the school.

This conclusion is in harmony with a view of the school's therapeutic potential arising from a secure, trusting, *teaching* relationship. The demands on the teacher, to pay close attention, to listen and respond to every child's initiative in a sympathetic way are immensely rewarded by the enhanced learning which can follow.

## Moving to Secondary School

The fact that moving from primary to secondary school is part of the normal life cycle for most children in Britain no doubt helps to reduce anxiety by making the transfer ordinary and anticipated well in advance. The magnitude of the change still means a period of considerable adjustment for most children and for some this produces difficulties which are not resolved in the process of settling down.

In the case of Susan transfer was complicated by absence for sickness in the first term at her large comprehensive school. She had transferred from a small, friendly primary school where she had made good average progress. The comprehensive school had a reputation for looking after its newcomers, but by the spring term she was reported to be falling behind in her work and to be intensely worried about this. Both the school staff and her parents expressed concern that they were not able to help her in spite of all their efforts at encouragement and support.

When seen at the clinic Susan's distress was very apparent and she was often close to tears. She described her problems in having no real friends, as all the children in her class had made up their friendship groups whilst she had been away. An especially important fact was that the only other girl from her 'old' school was in another class.

The theme of the previous primary school seemed especially important and was raised again in terms of Susan's envy of her younger sister who was still there. Encouraged to describe the school, she gave a highly idealised account of her time there and how happy she had been.

Invited to share her sense of loss, Susan revealed her intense grief, in spite of the fact that she had wanted to go to the particular comprehensive school she now attended. The mourning for her previous school eventually revealed its angry side also. This would be in line with accounts of grief and mourning and in Bowlby's attachment theory from which they derive, in which anger is identified as a normal component of grief.[8]

In Susan's case she produced an angry account of a bad memory when she had felt especially let down by a friend at the primary school. This had led her into quarrels with a group of her classmates not long before transfer. Following this discussion with the clinic psychologist, Susan brought reports of a much livelier engagement with other children in her present school. In this process of making alliances and having rows, Susan established some friendships and tackled an older girl who had been bullying her. In the clinic session in which she described this, she spoke of how the transfer to secondary school was like being at the bottom of the junior school again, and for the first time acknowledged that there too she had, in fact, needed to establish herself and make her own way. This also allowed her to consider the possibility of a more hopeful future and of change in her current position, and well before the end of the summer term her teachers reported her to be calmer and to be working better.

Looking back at her start in the secondary school Susan recalled in very concrete terms how lost she had then felt; rushing up and down stairs, not knowing which room to go to, feeling breathless and anxious.

Reminded of her sadness, too, at leaving her earlier school and how much harder it had been for her, because of her illness, to get over this, Susan agreed but said she no longer wanted to go back there, she was too grown up now.

Susan's subsequent progress in work and in social relationships was reported by her teachers to be very satisfactory, and there is no doubt that her own courage and determination were important factors in her adjustment. It seems likely that the problems which she highlighted are experienced by many other children. The focus of adjustment to the new school can obscure the need to give up the old one in a satisfactory way.

### Leaving School

This leads us to consideration of the last of these normal transitions, leaving school. There is a great deal of attention paid to preparation for those children moving on to further education. The examination system is geared to the selection needs of the universitites, and to some extent, the polytechnics too.

In an extended study of the way in which schools prepare their pupils to think about their future careers in work Scharff and Hill[9] reported on the problems of relating the subject matter of school to the world of work. In the research described, intense anxiety about the future was uncovered with a lack of effective strategies for coping with these anxieties.

The problems were intensified in the psychological milieu in which the actual event of leaving school took place. The children seemed to find difficulty in finding an adult who was effectively located at the point of transition between school and work. The orientation of the school staff was towards the world of school and this was being experienced by the youngsters going on to work as remote from the outside world they were about to enter.

The need to learn about work, rather than specific vocational preparation, is seen as the prerequisite for dealing with the crisis of the last year at school.

The psychological need to say goodbye in an effective and satisfying way gets lost in the tension of the last term, with its concentration on examinations and the usual gradual break up of the normal school week and a ragged drifting away from school.

### Career Choice

Career choice arouses intense anxiety among school leavers, and although this is recognised, too often discussion is based upon academic factors only, such as the child's best subjects at school, their general ability and, perhaps, a general look at their interests. Looking at other aspects is not to deny that the aforementioned attributes are relevant, but rather to draw attention to the emotional and psychological components of this process of choice and readiness for work.

The notion of readiness for school, socially, emotionally and intellectually has possibly been over stressed, especially as infant and nursery schools become more willing to adapt their methods to suit their newcomers. The notion of readiness for work is still undefined. Indeed those thrust first into the world of work are often amongst the least prepared. Whatever preparation there is, it is most often seen as a matter for the final year at school, with talks and lectures, careers exhibitions, maybe some vocational guidance questionnaires and visits to nearby factories, offices and so on.

To introduce these methods earlier, it is argued, is not meaningful to the young people themselves. This seems very likely to be true. Rather, it is a matter of looking at this sort of preparation in the last school year as just the culmination of a long process of growth towards the understanding of adult concepts which is, or should be, taking place throughout the years at secondary school. Independence and confidence, self awareness and an ability to survey one's own preferences and skills with some maturity are the kind of elements being referred to.

Such awareness includes the way in which feelings can be appropriately managed and brought under control, for the young person's investment in the choice made will be essential to its success and to a feeling of satisfaction.

**Examination Anxiety**

An example of the way in which even careful questionnaires and assessments can be misleading is provided by Peter. At 16 he was in considerable difficulties over his career choice. His best subject was mathematics, he disliked outdoor activity and he had an ability level rather above average. He was told that accountancy would be an ideal choice for him. However in subsequent discussions with the psychologist it became clear that Peter had a major difficulty with examinations, consistently failing to do himself real justice in them. To embark on a career based on such a sequence of exam hurdles as accountancy was useless without attention being paid to this problem. Either he required help with the causes of his examination difficulty or to choose a career in which they were much less important! Yet this original suggestion had followed a great deal of questionnaire type investigation.

The discovery of the emotional difficulty with examinations was further explored. Anxiety was linked not so much to a straightforward lack of belief in his own ability as in more complex interpersonal relationships, related especially to his father's expectations and his own reluctance to test himself out in an adult world.

Peter's maturity was not sufficient to equip him to be ready for career choice, although he was a well behaved and rather studious boy. Offering him techniques for managing examinations better was, in this context, to sidestep his need for time, and help, to mature, and therefore to leave his anxieties intact.

Adolescent striving for independence and recognition as a grown up is well recognised and indeed a frequent cause of rows at home. The fact that a youngster is not yet ready for complete independence is equally acknowledged. A less obvious contribution to the dilemma of growing up is the extent to which adolescents themselves may have a conflicting desire to remain dependent, and so safe and secure in childhood. Many occasions on which apparently well received advice fails may be accounted for by this underlying conflict. The more dependent a child seems the more likely we are to attempt to make decisions for him and the less opportunity we give him for developing the capacity to make his own.

## Other Transitions

Between these major transitions, of starting and leaving school, and of transfer from one school to another, is the yearly shift of class. This is so accepted that it is barely acknowledged as a source of anxiety at all. Such 'moving up' has, of course a positive side to it. In a way it stands for the school's acceptance that it is dealing with a population that is dynamic, changing and developing from year to year. The fact that this change of class is an essential part of school life undoubtedly also means that children expect it and are to some extent ready for it. An indirect reference to anxieties which are all the same close to the surface was contained in the comment of a headmaster who said that in his school no children were informed of the class they were to enter the following September until their first day back in school. His experience had been that raising the matter in the summer term led to too many requests, changing of minds, anxious letters from parents, and a general atmosphere of hysteria.

In another instance a teacher who had a friendly relationship with her primary school class shared with them the fact that she was leaving. This resulted in an enormous number of questions about her departure, but answering them did not reduce the amount of anxiety that she seemed to have aroused in the class. What the discussion subsequently appeared to give was an opportunity for the class to explore around the question of its own future. Who would they have next? What would the new teacher be like? Would he or she teach them in the same way? Such examples indicate how close to the surface such anxious questions are.

Allied to this is the special anxiety of the child joining a class after it has been established. Albert went to a new school a year after the main 11 + intake. He was keen to go to the school and looking forward to it. During the first term, however, he was failing to work as well as anticipated. He was a sociable boy and the difficulty which might be expected of making friends when friendship groups have already been formed did not seem to be a special problem for him. On interview he revealed his considerable concern with trying to understand 'the rules'. The school itself did not consider that it had an especially rigid structure or a large number of fixed rules. What Albert spoke of were the customs and habits which the other children had by now acquired. For him the lack of definite school rules was no help, rather the contrary. Learning where things were kept, who to go to, how to get new books and many other things, including much apparently trivial detail, filled his day.

The effort he had to make to pick things up is not so noticeable when a whole class is new. It is worth noting all the same as a feature of all transitions. The need for quite detailed information is clear, but the attempt to give this too quickly only seems to result in it not being taken in. The experience for the teachers can be frustrating if they are not themselves prepared to make allowance for the emotional aspects of being a newcomer with its associated feelings of bewilderment and uncertainty.

It is suggested that the process of 'settling in' requires thought at every transition. For a minority of children the process is not achieved because chances are lost at the moment of transfer, and a foundation laid for future school problems.

## Anxieties about Learning

The causes of learning difficulties and the debates about dyslexia, IQs and remedial programmes are important but the intention here is to look rather at the anxieties about learning which may not necessarily be associated with actual failure.

Again, working with individual children can shed light on the nature of the anxieties and may, it is hoped, therefore be of help to the many children for whom such individual counselling is not possible.

The technique of educational therapy is especially useful in this respect since it pays particular attention to the emotional aspects of the learning difficulty, alongside careful teaching of the actual skills involved. The technique is fully described in Caspari[10] but the interest here is in the understanding of the child's relationship to the teacher/therapist on which it is based. The importance of cognitive factors and of good teaching is not denied but, implicit in all such good teaching is the relationship in which it takes place.

The feelings are expressed through games and expressive materials. In this way negative aspects of the relationship may be given an outlet without undermining the predominantly positive mood that the teacher encourages. Rivalry with the adult may be safely encouraged through a competitive game, and if the child wins the teacher is pleased.

The type of destruction of an opponent which ends a competitive game is acceptable to both sides, guilty feelings are kept within bounds and anxieties can be contained. Anxieties about losing and failing, cheating and changing the rules can be dealt with in a real way but at one remove from the crucial situation of the classroom itself.

Sometimes, however, even games are too direct in the feelings they arouse and other types of expression work, painting, drawing, modelling and story telling may allow negative and anxious feelings to be revealed and discussed at one remove. The child may identify with the emotions of his/her characters, but this identification need not be revealed. An attack on another character may be linked with a wished for attack on family or friend but it is kept within the bounds of the picture or story.

Sessions with children in which feelings are encouraged to be expressed in this way reveal the immense importance attached to the teacher's reliability and constancy. The fact that more hostile and aggressive feelings can be included in an indirect way prevents a cosy one to one situation in which progress is based upon idealisation of the teacher.

The importance of avoiding such idealisation cannot be overestimated, since the perfection it presupposes can never in fact be realised. Moreover the relationship must come to an end and the effect then can be to arouse bitter feelings of rejection in the child which lead in turn to rejection of the learning associated with the teacher.

Within the classroom the focus on the subject matter of the teaching may contain a similar possibility for much indirect expression and containment of feelings. In another article Caspari[11] discusses in an imaginative and original way, the contribution which the ordinary curriculum can make to the management of anxieties.

Taking as her starting point the relationship between teacher and pupil she quotes Winnicott.[12] His view was that the school situation gives the child a special opportunity to come to terms with emotional conflicts via a relationship with an adult, the teacher, which is intense yet less emotionally charged than relationships at home.

Although Winnicott was referring to nursery age children, Caspari suggests that this remains true for older children also. Within this relationship it is important that expression be given to the negative feelings aroused even in a good relationship, by the need to do things the child does not like or want to do at that moment. The expression of such feelings needs, however, to be done in an acceptable way, hence games and expression work.

So far this approach is very much like that of the individual educational therapy described above. What Caspari goes on to point out is the contribution made by the subject. Literature is the clearest example, and I can recall how a gifted teacher of English managed by skilful choice of reading to guide her class in discussion through many of the most sensitive issues for adolescents. Essay writing, history, geography and all the lessons which give an opportunity to look at the lives and feelings of other people are appropriate to this approach. Equally interesting are the opportunities offered by other, more abstract subjects. Caspari quotes the case of mathematics and how teaching a child to do his own checking back was a way of handing to him some of the feeling of control which he so desperately needed. It began a process of sorting out what could be controlled and what could not which was very valuable to him.

## Anxieties about Going to School

A final word needs to be said about the greatest anxiety of all about school, which results in a refusal to attend.

This has been discussed in many places and a summary of the thinking about 'school phobia' is contained in Kahn, Nursten and Carroll.[13] It points to the difference between truancy and school phobia, which is based on acute anxiety which persists even though both child and parents want him/her to go to school. It is now often assumed therefore that the problem lies at home rather than at school, in fact that the anxiety is concerned with leaving home, and it is not unusual to hear teachers say that the child is quite all right once settled in class. However, Kahn *et al.* point out that the term 'school phobia' has become an umbrella term which covers many different forms of difficulty. Fear of school may be present, although it may be transferred or displaced from home. A change of school may only result in a new focus being chosen.

The interrelationship of home and school factors is illustrated in the case of a 6-year-old girl, Clare, who was refusing to go to school after absence due to a bout of influenza. This is a not uncommon time for such refusal to appear for the first time, and, as is also often the case, attempts to persuade her led to her becoming quite frantic.

Psychological assessment suggested a preoccupation with aggressive themes which was at odds with Clare's sweet appearance. Her history revealed a good deal of feeding difficulty, originating with breast feeding which had been disturbed for a number of unavoidable reasons. In her drawings and stories the target of the oral aggression (biting animals and dead, half devoured creatures) was confused. Curiosity led to damage and destruction and yet powerful figures were both envied and dangerous.

The difficulty in leaving her mother was clearly related by

Clare to her anxieties about what would happen to her mother while she was at school. What only later became clear was the extent of her own hostile feelings to her mother and Clare's own need to protect both herself and her mother from this hostility. The feelings instead, were related to the teacher at school, but a further important factor was the danger inherent in the learning situation itself. Finding out was felt by Clare not to be safe. There were also many positive aspects to Clare, of course. Her wish to make amends for damage, her ability to function well when she felt safe could be built upon and a return to school was successfully achieved over the next few months.

## Summary

This chapter draws many of its examples from clinical experience but the main concern is with children who come within a normal range rather than the deeply anxious or disturbed child.

The contribution that the school makes to anxiety is related in particular to the way in which transitions are handled, especially starting and leaving school. Other anxieties related more specifically to the learning situation are examined and brief reference made to the complexities which lie behind the blanket description 'school phobia'.

## References

1. Robertson, J., *Young Children in Hospital*, 2nd edn (Tavistock Publications, London, 1970).

2. Bowlby, J., 'A Control Systems Approach to Attachment Behaviour', in *Attachment and Loss*, vol. 1, Chapter 13 (Hogarth Press, London, 1969).

3. Ainsworth, M. D. S., Blehar, M. C., Waters, E. and Wall, S., *Patterns of Attachment: A Psychological Study of the Strange Situation* (Lawrence Erlbaum Associates, Hillsdale, New Jersey, 1978).

4. Blatchford, P., Battle, S. and Mays, J., *The First Transition: Home to Pre-School* (NFER-Nelson, Windsor, 1982).

5. Janis, M. G., *A Two-Year-Old Goes to Nursery School: A Case Study of Separation Reactions* (Tavistock Publications, London, 1964).

6. Holmes, E., 'The Effectiveness of Educational Intervention for Pre-school Children in Day and Residential Care', *New Growth, 2(1),* (1982), pp. 17–30.

7. Cleave, S. Jowett, S. and Bate, M., *And So To School: A Study of Continuity from Pre-School to Infant School* (NFER-Nelson, Windsor, 1982).

8. Boxall, M., *The Nurture Group in the Primary School* (ILEA, 1976).

9. Scharff, D. E. and Hill, J., *Between Two Worlds: Aspects of the Transition from School to Work* (London Careers Consultants Ltd, 1976).

10. Caspari, I., 'Educational Therapy' in V. Varma (ed.), *Psychotherapy Today* (Constable, London, 1974).

11. Caspari, I., *The Curriculum: Emotional Stability, The Contribution of the Curriculum.* Reprint from Conference Speeches held at Queen Elizabeth Hall, London, 1970.

12. Winnicott, D. M., *The Child and the Outside World* (Tavistock Publications, London, 1957).

13. Kahn, J. H., Nursten, J. P. and Carroll, H. C. M., *Unwillingly to School*, 3rd edn (Pergamon Press, Oxford, 1981).

# 10 ANXIETY RELATING TO ILLNESS AND TREATMENT

Lindy Burton

This chapter deals with the anxieties created for children by illness and treatment experiences. An attempt is made to relate such fears to the child's age and level of maturity at the time of the experience, and to the emotional climate which surrounds him. The nature of his symptoms, the presence of pain, and the type of treatment required will also be related to the kinds of fears he may sustain. Whilst much work in this area has resulted from sympathetic assessments of chronically ill or dying children, some studies relate only to generally well children and an attempt will be made to distinguish between the anxieties created for each group.

**Introduction: A Case Study**

A 19-year-old undergraduate came to me recently for counselling. She reported difficulties in making and sustaining relationships, and in persevering with her academic studies. Looking at her, I saw a bright cheerful, good-looking girl, whose educational attainments I knew to be excellent, certainly not the sort of girl one would have expected to experience such problems. Upon investigation, she admitted to feeling inadequate, vulnerable, and somehow damaged. She was worried about her ability to pass her final exams, and she doubted her ability to sustain her present emotional commitment. Exploration of these feelings revealed that periodically she sustained a very frightening nightmare. In this she felt herself to be crippled, and actually saw herself in a wheelchair, completely immobilised, and utterly alone. Whilst restrained in this way, she sensed, and became deeply afraid of, something or someone approaching. She knew she was about to be hurt or maimed in some way, and yet she was powerless to escape. Normally at this point in the nightmare she awoke, terrified. Even recalling the dream elicited noticeable emotion, yet at first she was unable to explain the dream content. Only after protracted questioning did she reveal that she had once been ill and hospitalised. She added, almost dismissively, that it was a very long time ago! She was three years old at the time, and had required surgery for appendicitis. She could still remember being rushed into hospital in a friend's car, being almost forcibly separated from her mother, and being prepared for an operation for which she was given no pre-medication.

As she talked, my client began to recollect the terror she had experienced when faced with a ring of huge, gowned figures, all standing around waiting to do something to her. She remembered being held down on an operating table, whilst someone put a mask over her face. Although she struggled, it had proved impossible to escape. Later, recovering in a vast, shiny ward, she had screamed and screamed, not just from loneliness, but because she was convinced that somehow they had changed her in some way. She could not remember anyone talking to her, or anyone reassuring her about the operation. Presumably, at that time, those caring for her still believed that she was too small to need or benefit from such consolation.

The significance of these recollections in terms of this young woman's later emotional and educational difficulties needs little explanation. Like so many other small children subjected to unexplained and often frightening illness and treatment procedures, she had evolved a fantasy in which her surgery had subtly but permanently damaged her. This fantasy was strengthened, rather than diminished, by the additional pampering she received from her parents on return home. Their solicitousness and cossetting somehow added to her sense of violation and vulnerability, and this was so pervasive that it lasted unresolved throughout her childhood, colouring not only her self image, but also much of her behaviour.

### Anxiety Observed in the Behaviour of Generally Well Behaved Children

One would like to believe that this young woman was unique, but common sense and careful observation suggest otherwise. Although most hospital staff are now extremely sensitive to the emotional needs of their young patients, and many units have devised elegant systems of preparation,[1] and patient support, even routine, and minimal illness and treatment procedures can cause anxiety.[2-8] Such anxiety can be expressed in many ways. Some fears are verbalised either directly or obliquely. Other fears are expressed behaviourally. Many children, hospitalised for quite minor procedures look scared, become agitated, breathe deeply, tremble, stop talking or playing, and even start to cry when treatment time arrives. Others unexpectedly wet or soil themselves, and some actively attempt to escape from the grasp of those who are trying to help them. This is especially noticeable if the child believes the treatment will be painful, or if it has not been fully explained, and he fears it will be unpleasant or beyond his ability to cope.

From the child's standpoint, fight or flight behaviours subserve several functions. First they attract attention to the child's distress, and are therefore useful in terms of alerting others to his need for additional emotional support. Second, they give the child some sense of control in the situation, thereby diminishing a damaging sense of helplessness.

### Anxiety Observed in the Behaviour of Chronically Sick Children

Not all children express their anxiety so openly, however. Some chronically ill children, who have become accustomed to illness and treatment procedures appear almost indifferent to all that is happening. This is not to say their illness experiences do not frighten them, quite the reverse. Many are apprehensive and depressed, but familiarity with procedures and staff diminishes their need to display anxiety in any organised or obvious way. Instead they may communicate their fears by subtly changed emotional states, by becoming moody and cross[9-11] or inexplicably non-verbal. Some unexpectedly protest at, or repudiate, treatment, or become acutely angry in the face of other, unexpected and trivial health care requirements, for example going to the dentist.[12] Some children play or draw out their fantasies,[13,14] or tell or write stories centring on illness themes.[12,15-17] Others express their fears in dreams.[18] Very small children may become more dependent, more babyish, and subject to night terrors.[12] At all ages sleeping difficulties may suddenly emerge, the child seeming unwilling or afraid to fall asleep.

In many cases illness-related anxieties colour the child's approach to general social and educational contacts. Spina bifida children are described as passive, lacking in drive, fearing inferiority, and fearful of new things.[17] Children with cystic fibrosis are often afraid of new tasks and strange situations, and timid with people.[12] As with asthmatic children[19] they often defend themselves from people and situations which they fear will be too stressful for them. Many sick children have an envy, almost a fantasy about their normal peers, thinking of them as perfect.[17]

### The Anxiety of Sick Children. A Challenge to Those Who Care for the Sick Child

Faced with such manifest indices of anxiety one would presume that all paediatricians, nurses and parents would be making heroic efforts to combat the emotional distress of sick children in their care. Sadly, this does not always happen. Whilst some have evolved most excellent caring strategies to keep the child emotionally 'secure',[20-25] others seem not to notice even obvious emotional pain.

Unwillingness to acknowledge a child's emotional distress may occur for many reasons. Sometimes doctors, nurses, and even parents are too overburdened by the physical tasks which face them to have time or energy to grapple with the child's more intangible emotional needs. Occasionally, adult care givers themselves find the implications of the child's illness too emotionally challenging to undertake anything other than direct physical care. This is especially true where the child's illness is life threatening, or involves a great reduction in overall functioning. Hospital units which regularly care for dying children, and which have no staff support systems, may be especially disadvantaged in this respect. Constant exposure to the anxiety of sick children is very threatening, and young, inexperienced, or insecure staff may be too anguished themselves to acknowledge the child's fears directly, defending themselves instead by providing unremitting physical care. This in turn taxes and tires them, reducing even further their ability to cope with a child's fears.

Sometimes, in the case of seriously ill children, the adult care giver may be so challenged professionally by his inability to reverse disease, that gradually he is forced to withdraw from the child. As a result he will distance himself emotionally, and sometimes even physically from such a child.[15,24-28] Parents can experience similar feelings. Those who are least secure may find their child's illness so threatening that they are forced to defend themselves by denying at least some of its significance. In the process they become less sensitive to the child's emotional needs.[24] Thus many sick children are forced to bear their illness fears and fantasies without the emotional support of those close to them. Understandably emotional isolation can potentiate a child's fear.[29,30] Perhaps what is needed in all these cases is a willingness on the adult's part to acknowledge his limitations, and to seek help from someone who is willing, and able, to support the child emotionally. In the larger Children's Hospitals the team generally involves a child psychologist, or children's social worker, who is able to undertake this task. Similarly such help is available in the community through the psychology and social work departments of local authorities.

**Coping with Illness-Related Anxiety**

How do illness fears arise, and how can those who care for the sick child best meet his emotional needs?

There is no easy answer to this question. Each child is unique, and events which affect one adversely may present little undue difficulty for another. Each child must be assessed very thoroughly. His unique personality, with its strengths, weaknesses and coping strategies must be considered. Also one must take account of the support he receives from those closest to him. In addition, one must consider the exact illness circumstances, whether the illness necessitates hospitalisation or treatment, produces frightening, disfiguring, or embarrassing symptoms, or pain, has a good or poor prognosis, all these circumstances govern the fears which may arise.

In addition, those of us who are called upon to support the child emotionally must take account of the child's age and maturational status. The degree and type of anxiety produced by illness varies greatly dependent on the child's level of emotional, social, and intellectual maturity. It is also influenced by the child's perception of the feeling tone of others. Even if the child is not inherently frightened by what is happening to him, he may learn to fear because of subtle changes in the behaviour of others towards him.

**Fears Dependent on a Sick Child's Age and Level of Maturity**

Generally childhood is a time in which the growing individual acquires all the skills necessary for separate adult life. During his development a child gradually relinquishes his total dependence on others, and begins to develop a sense of self reliance, based on his own ability to explore, manipulate, and eventually master his environment. To fulfil his potential the child needs constant opportunities and consistent encouragement to try out new skills. Also he requires continual protection from trauma, which may diminish his courage and willingness to develop.

Illness, and treatment, which so frequently deprive the child of freedom, a sense of independence, and the opportunities to explore and experiment[5,31,32] negates these strivings for self expression, and are therefore deeply disorientating. This is true for all children, whether generally well, or chronically ill. Naturally the more protracted the illness and treatment experiences, the more threatening they will be. One must therefore assess the extent and nature of the procedures involved when one assesses the resultant fears. Similarly one must consider the child's age and level of maturity.

For the infant there is no threat in being nursed and tended by another. On the contrary, total dependence is normal at this age, and essential for survival. Illness should not therefore disorientate an infant, provided he is cared for by a familiar adult, preferably in a familiar environment.

Problems arise if infants are faced with unfamiliarity for, example, transferral to hospital with consequent changes in routine. Even the youngest infant responds adversely to such moves, senses differences in handling, feeding and changing.[12,33] For this reason mothers of ailing infants should be encouraged to retain care of their children, whether at home or in hospital.

During the pre-school period the young child's relationship with his parents becomes increasingly intense. They are his principal source of physical satisfaction, and his safe haven in times of distress. In addition, because they usually encourage and provide opportunities for the gradual unfolding of his abilities, they become crucial for the development of his skills.

Illness, if it entails separation from them, and handling by others is therefore a fundamental threat at many different levels.[34-37] As with the infant therefore, if illness necessitates hospitalisation, every care should be taken to keep the pre-school child and his parents together. Separation is the real fear at this age, not physical decline, or even death, and separation anxiety is avoidable if the help of parents is properly elicited.[6,21,22,33,35,38-42]

When a young child is suddenly, inexplicably deprived of the comfort and support of those closest to him, he may exhibit the classic syndrome of protest, withdrawal, and despair.[34] In the final analysis this separation may lead him to feel unloved and unlovable, and if the separation is compounded by frightening, unexplained treatments, he may believe himself to be permanently damaged, and these feelings may permeate his whole existence for years afterwards, as in the case of the young student described above.

The ability to tend to oneself at the toilet, to wash, dress, eat and drink unaided are all fundamental skills, acquired painstakingly by all children, whether generally well or chronically sick. None of these attributes is surrendered lightly, and children of all ages protest vehemently against yielding control over them. This is especially true of pre-school children, whose sense of self is rooted in personal control of physical functions. Every sick child whether at home or in hospital, should therefore be encouraged to do as much as possible for himself.[43] This helps the child to feel active and independent, and reminds him that his illness is only relative, and that he still possesses many intact faculties. By contrast, where children have to surrender control of their basic skills unnecessarily, they often become unnecessarily passive, depressed, and begin to doubt their own abilities.[17]

Naturally, school-age children will have learnt to separate from their parents, and will be used to strange environments and contacts with unfamiliar adults. If illness necessitates hospitalisation their more-developed social skills will enable them to adjust, at least if they have been properly prepared for the event,[1] and are accompanied by parents during the settling in phase. Some more generally apprehensive children, perhaps children who have already sustained separation anxiety for other reasons, or children who appear inherently timorous, may still have problems in adapting to hospital care, however, and need special support if they are not to sustain further separation anxiety with consequent physical decline.[12,36]

One of the major problems facing seriously ill school age children is that almost invariably illness limits the number of things they can do. Whether at home or in hospital, illness is often accompanied by a sense of boredom, and this contributes to feelings of inadequacy and worthlessness.[17,36,44,45] To counteract this, all sick children need as rich and demanding a life as possible.[23] Purposeful school work should be recommenced as soon as children can cope with it, for school work not only fills empty hours, but also gives the child a sense of achievement, and some hope for the future.[21,46–48] Hospital schools, necessary even in short-stay units, are crucial in long-stay establishments, and home tuition is essential for the child who is confined to the home. In addition, sick children should be encouraged to be as mobile as possible, playing and living each day as fully as they can. Such freedom and encouragement will maintain their sense of personal worth and diminish self doubts.

Although separation is the paramount fear of small children, pain, difigurement, inadequacy, and ultimate unacceptability are the essential fears of older children.[2–6,12,17,29,49–54] Some of these fears spring from inadequately explained, and therefore inadequately understood, treatment procedures, some from the fantasies which the child weaves concerning his illness. All sick children have such fears, though chronically ill, and dying children are especially disadvantaged, often gradually changing their self images to accord with the changes which they perceive in the behaviour of those around them.

As with the fears of younger children, amelioration of these fears is essential for the older child's emotional survival. Like the adult, he needs to know that he is acceptable to others despite his illness, and that he is valuable. In order to have the courage to face up to his physical difficulties, he must believe there is a place for him in the world. If sick children can be encouraged to believe this, rather than becoming disheartened and depressed, many will develop additional skills to compensate for their inadequacies. Chronically sick children frequently become more verbal, more sympathetic to others, and often have a sustaining sense of humour.[12,16] Some show greater fastidiousness in dress and personal appearance, and, if they possess special talents, work hard to maximise these.[45,50,51,55,56] In this way the chronically sick child. who is properly supported, manages to contain and use his anxieties positively.

One of the most taxing problems with older children is that some of them do equate serious illness with death. As a result they may become genuinely concerned for their own mortality. Sometimes such fears are prompted by subtle changes in the behaviour of others towards them, and occasionally they arise from the cruel taunts of other children.[49] In some instances it is the death of another child with the same disease, either met on the ward, or in the outpatient clinic, which triggers off such fears, especially if these deaths are hastily and clumsily denied.[11,26,57]

Although it has been known for children as young as three to voice fears of death,[58] generally, the younger child's notions concerning this state are confused and sketchy, death being equated with the more fundamental age-appropriate fears of abandonment and separation. By mentioning death, very young children are usually seeking reassurance that they will not be left alone. Older sick children, or children with lengthy illness experiences, are a great deal more sophisticated, however. Even as early as five or six they may begin to appreciate the finality of death[26,59] and fear that their illness will result in their own demise. Often sick children equate death with pain, violence, and burial in dark places. They are understandably distressed. Seriously ill teenage patients are especially sensitive in this respect and their fears of personal extinction may become such that, in order to contain them, they are forced to pretend that they are not really ill. For this reason some chronically ill children may suddenly and unexpectedly repudiate their treatment programmes. Some children with cystic fibrosis,[12,60] diabetes[61] and multiple sclerosis[55] manifest such behaviour. Unconsciously they argue that if they do not have treatment, they do not have disease, and in an effort to defend themselves against the emotional implications of their disease they refuse further medication. Children in this state are obviously at greater risk from illness.

Clearly, in the interests of the older child's physical and emotional well being, absolute denial of this sort cannot be allowed to persist. Whilst intermittent denial is probably an effective means of coping with illness-related fears, gross denial is undoubtedly disruptive. What one should aim for, I believe, is a situation in which the chronically sick child feels secure enough to admit that he has a physical disability, which requires regular treatment, but at the same time is determined to lead as normal a life as possible. If he can forget his illness, between treatment times, so much the better.

## Fears which Mirror the Emotional Discomfort of Others

Generally sick children are least anxious when those they love and trust remain accepting and supportive in the face of their illness. If parents, siblings, and close friends see the child's affliction as relative, remain cheerful and optimistic, and are not themselves discomforted by the illness circumstances, then the sick child's anxiety is lessened. Sadly the reverse is also true. Where parents are embarrassed, anxious or depressed, as often happens when the illness is obvious, or the diagnosis serious, then their attitudes convey themselves quickly to the child, who in turn becomes emotionally discomforted.[7,22,29,37,62,63] Often very little is actually said, parents being too distressed to face the matter openly, but nonetheless the child detects and mirrors his parents' feelings. Diffidence and withdrawal, sighs, lingering unhappy looks, even sudden unexpected presents, all alert the child to the presence of something to be feared.[64] Obviously such fears are exaggerated where parents markedly change in their expectations for, and handling of, their sick child. If they make unnecessary differences between him and his siblings this will add to his worries.[65] Even subtle changes in their mood may disturb him. Infants also are sensitive to their mother's feelings. By a process of contagion they seem to absorb and reflect their mother's moods.

All those surrounding the sick child should be challenged to treat him as normally as possible, to accord him respect for his intact faculties, and provide him with the opportunities for play and self expression. Not only will this combat his fears, but it will help them.

## Fears Relating to a Sick Child's Symptoms

Infants and pre-school children are essentially egotistical, and rarely compare themselves with others. As a result they normally accept their symptoms, however gross, without undue upset.[43] Exceptions to this rule are found, however, in families where the parents themselves are so distressed by these symptoms that they become acutely anxious and communicate their own anxiety directly or indirectly to the child.[12,49] In such cases apprehension may be conveyed even by a mother's unwillingness to touch or handle an affected area. In such cases, the pre-school child who responds with anxiety is usually responding more to his parents' feelings than to actual disease manifestations. Generally, it is not until the child emerges from the age of egocentricity and starts

comparing himself with well brothers and sisters, or intact school-
mates, that he develops genuine discomfort concerning his
symptoms. Obviously the way in which he responds to these will
largely depend upon their exact nature and the degree to which they
interfere with the gradual unfolding of his abilities, similarly, the
way in which others view the symptoms will shape the child's own
response to them. Where symptoms are very obvious and disfiguring, the child may feel unacceptable to others, and respond with
shame and embarrassment, especially if he is met with aversion or
fear.[17] This is especially true of children whose illness has a late
onset and who have not therefore spent pre-school years accommo-
dating to their disability. Where this happens, a child may become
afraid in social circumstances, and, unless help is given, he may tend
to become isolated and solitary. Care should be taken constantly to
praise such children concerning their other intact faculties. Even
grossly deformed children can make some accommodation to their
handicap if handled with sufficient sensitivity.[45]

Where symptoms are less obvious, but ever present, as in the case
of many chronic conditions, they may be resented because they
prevent full participation in normal play or classroom activities.
This both isolates the child and contributes to his growing sense of
'difference'. Parents can help to counteract the upset this
engenders by assisting the child's conformity in other ways, for
example, by providing the 'right' clothes, school equipment, or
hair do.

Teenage children often worry that their symptoms will prevent
them obtaining, or holding down, a job. These fears can be eased
by parents sympathetically investigating the employment situation
or taking the child to a Careers Advisory Centre, which should
provide information concerning suitable job opportunities.

Where symptoms are not fully understood, or emerge unexpectedly, they may produce considerable fear in parents and children.
Wherever possible, both should be warned in advance of their
probable occurrence. Similarly, both should be assured that
nothing they did, or omitted to do, contributed to the development
of such symptoms. It is not unusual for parents and children to feel
vaguely responsible, and even guilty, for the emergence of
symptoms unless proper explanations have been given.

Occasionally parents and children assess physical progress with
reference to symptoms, using them as a barometer by which to
judge the child's overall health. Anxiety concerning symptoms may

therefore represent anxiety concerning the overall illness, just as protest about symptoms, or treatment, may mask more fundamental fears. Often a child who worries or protests in such ways is expressing his fears of loneliness, difference, worthlessness, or death, in a manner that he knows will be acceptable to others. He knows that his parents or nurses will tolerate upsets concerning symptoms, or treatments, and endeavour to comfort him as a result, whereas he senses, often rightly, that they may become apprehensive and withdrawn if he asks for reassurance for his more fundamental fears.[17,66]

Whatever the negative aspects of symptoms, at least they do indicate that the disease is present, and children displaying them can be treated as if they are ill. In this sense their lot is easier than that of some other seriously ill children who may lack obvious or easily discernible manifestations of their condition. Having no way of monitoring changes in their state, they are left with the constant fear that they are deteriorating. In such cases some children become overly self absorbed, anxiously scrutinising themselves for supposed changes in well being, rigorously guarding themselves against minimal physical hardship.[53]

An apparent lack of obvious symptoms can be especially disorientating at the outset of an illness, contributing as it often does to delay in diagnosis, with consequent parental upset. Sometimes, in the early stages of an illness, ephemeral changes in the child's well being may be misconstrued as naughtiness and punishment may be given. Occasionally even seriously ill children have been taken to Child Guidance Clinics for assessment and counselling before it was realised that they were actually physically ill. Such experiences invariably cloud the child's attitude to his illness, making him feel guilty and bad because of it. Occasionally his relationship with his parents is also undermined. In turn such experiences may add to the parents' sense of guilt, and their feelings of inadequacy in dealing with the disease will subtly convey themselves to the child, further eroding his ability to come to terms with his illness.

Where a disease continues without markedly obvious symptomatology it may be difficult for parents to really believe that it exists, and to ensure that the child receives necessary treatment. Similarly they may encounter difficulties because the illness is not taken seriously by their friends or family. Their consequent sense of social discomfort and isolation may rebound on the sick child, adding to his sense of difference.

## Fears Related to Pain

Pain is not conducive to well being at any age, yet despite this our attitudes to it are fundamentally confused.[5,6,31,59] This is especially true of our attitudes to pain in children. Even today some who care for young children deny that they experience such discomfort, or that such feelings are of significance in terms of their adaptation to disease. But this is not the case. Even infants show evidence of pain, although their response to it is gross, rather than discrete. With increasing age, a child's ability to report and detect pain, improves. He is better able to indicate its site, and to seek comfort for it. He may be no more stoical in the face of it however, and, like the small child, he may fantasise that it has come as a punishment for something he did or failed to do, or that it is part of some corrosive internal process which will undoubtedly destroy him. Many children confuse the original pain with subsequent attempts to alleviate it, and this further feeds fantasies of being punished or destroyed.[5] Physical pain should never be allowed to persist. Every attempt should be made to alleviate it.[31,59]

## Fears and Anxieties Associated with Treatment

Many factors contribute to the way in which a sick child views his treatment. As with his response to illness generally, age and level of maturity are important considerations.[67] So also are the nature of the treatments, and the extent to which they affect his sense of physical well being. Additionally the attitude of his parents, siblings, and peers towards his treatment is crucial.

Generally children have fewer fears when their treatment regime is commenced in infancy and becomes part of the unvarying routine of their everyday life. In such cases sick children have habituated to the treatment long before they are prompted to question its significance. Obviously the nature of the treatment is important in this respect, taking tablets and medicines to stay well is more usual and less disruptive of play than treatments such as postural drainage or physiotherapy. Tablet taking is therefore tolerated better by children of all ages.[12] Similarly, if care is taken from the outset to make the treatment task as pleasant as possible, it will be less frightening. If parents take the trouble to explain why the therapy is needed, and if they couple it with conversation and play, it will produce less discomfort.

With older children, especially those diagnosed beyond infancy, treatment may be disliked and feared because it becomes a symbol of the child's illness, accentuating his sense of difference from others,[12,55,60,61] Naturally, the more obvious the therapy, the more equipment involved, the less the child can disguise it, the more socially discomforting it will become. Older children may need an opportunity to express their distress, and to become better informed concerning the nature and usefulness of the required regimes. Some parents may lack the ability to talk over such matters, either because they do not know the facts, or because they are afraid of frightening or hurting the child by voicing the subject.[16] In such circumstances another caring adult should be appointed to discuss the treatment regime with the child. He may be helped in this task if provided beforehand with one of the excellent manuals for young patients now being provided to explain complicated treatment procedures.[68]

Some treatment procedures undoubtedly have punitive overtones, for example, those requiring bedrest, or immobilisation,[6,53,69] swallowing unpleasant substances, isolation[69] or a limitation of food intake. Understandably, some children faced with such treatments see them as evidence of rejection, or view them as punishment for wrong doing, perhaps as a dreadful adult retaliation for becoming sick.[5,58] Such children need reassurance about these fears, especially concerning any sense of guilt or responsibility they may have. In extreme cases perceptual and bodily disturbances and acute loss of identity may be found in children whose treatment demands physical isolation.[16,52] Great care must be taken to maintain verbal and emotional contact with such children, and reassurance must be given that the treatment is only for their good, and that it will be discontinued as quickly as possible.[70] Sometimes children placed in physical isolation misconstrue the situation, believing that they are placed apart for the sake of others, rather than for their own sake. Such thoughts should be watched for, and banished, before they assume frightening proportions.

Even a home-based treatment programme may have its dangers, for example, occasionally, it may make parents feel over responsible for the sick child's ultimate survival. As a result, some become over zealous in administering the therapy. Focusing their whole attention on this aspect of their child's existence. When this happens the child's wider social, emotional, and intellectual needs may be neglected.[9,61] The child is thus deprived of a full existence, made more anxious for his own safety, and encouraged to become over dependent on his parents.[25,71,72] This in turn discourages his strivings for independence and tends to increase his underlying anxiety. If at any time he becomes temporarily stronger he may protest against the arrangement, repudiating the treatment.[62] Such protests, unless properly understood, may frighten parents and child alike, alienating one from the other.

Casual observers often think that children kept on treatment for a long time must eventually adapt to it, so that in the end they accept it without apprehension. This is rarely the case, especially when treatment procedures are unpleasant, causes discomfort, or interrupt normal life. In such circumstances children continually and understandably endeavour to evade them. In this context parental attitudes are of enormous importance. Any weakness on the parents' part, or hesitation in giving therapy, is quickly recognised and exploited by the child. The child may argue that the treatment hurts, or makes him feel sick, or he is tired or fed up. Insecure parents, unable to accept their child's hostility,[73] or parents who have been insufficiently counselled regarding the need for treatment, may crumble in the face of these protests. As a result, the child will probably increase his manipulations, with a consequent increase in his parents' inconsistency. Only an unremitting positive approach to therapy will do, and before this can be achieved, parents must not only be fully cognisant of how to give the therapy, but also understand the reasons for its use.

The obviousness of the survival value of the treatment for the child is a further factor affecting his feelings towards it. Generally, when a child really needs treatment he will respond best to it. Similarly, children whose treatment has markedly improved their well being are less fearful of it subsequently.

As previously stressed, infants and young children with little standard of comparison seem to adapt best to alterations in life style necessitated by treatment. By contrast, the older the child is at the onset of his illness, the greater has been his previous freedom, the harder it is for him to accept the limitations imposed by treatment.[31,43] The more limiting the procedures, the more exacting is this adaptation.[6,53] Consequently, children with severe disabilities requiring bedrest, immobilisation, or confinement to a wheelchair often use all their self control in maintaining a superficially accepting attitude. When additional stress is placed upon them, especially if this emanates from domestic rather than medical sources, such children frequently react with what appears, from a distance, to be excessive emotion.[18] Simple changes in domestic routine trigger off temper tantrums, visits to the dentist prompt angry scenes, family quarrels produce disproportionate despair. It is as if the child is already so heavily burdened that he cannot tolerate any additional stress. Naturally, this makes the task of caring for such children an additionally complex one. Any change must be introduced gradually, with as much preparation and warning as possible. Parents must be advised of the need for consistency in their handling of the child, yet at the same time, they must be aided in devising a management plan which emphasises 'normality' and not damaging compensatory overprotection.[18,74] It is surprising how often even the most sensible parents become pamperers in the face of their sick child's protests. But pampering rarely produces any marked improvement in the child's behaviour, rather it increases his confusion and level of anxiety, and often results in growing resentment and discord on the part of less-indulged siblings.

## Defences Against Illness-induced Anxiety

Most children are challenged emotionally by their illness and treatment. Whether generally well, or chronically sick, some may feel lessened or violated because of illness experiences. As a result, they may doubt their acceptability to others, and wonder whether they are really lovable. Insecurity and apprehension may result.

Not all sick children are overwhelmed by anxiety, however. Some not only emerge from the experience emotionally unscathed, but even appear strengthened as a result. Careful observation of this phenomenon led Jessner[75] to comment: 'Illness may not only spur maturation, but also widen the horizon, heighten sensitivity, bring forth a greater depth of feeling, capacity for empathy and sublimation.' Further observation has shown that sick children can show sustaining humour, and great courage,[12] and some work extra hard to develop skills,[76] or take greater care of their appearance in order to compensate for their disability.[51,56]

Even severely ill children can transcend the apprehensions caused by their illness experiences. For example, Morrisey[58] working with leukaemic children, found that 70 per cent made a good overall adjustment to hospitalisation despite severe or noticeable anxiety. He commented: 'Two children may have similar levels of anxiety, but the anxiety may operate differently in the two individuals, one child may be emotionally paralysed, the other one use resources constructively to keep anxiety under control.'

Similarly Tropauer *et al.*[51] working with children with cystic fibrosis, commented: 'It is not the existence of anxiety *per se* that handicaps the sick child and intensifies his invalidism, but rather its degree and his methods of dealing with it.'

Very little is known about the processes by which children transcend their illness experience. Rosenstein[72] emphasises the usefulness of the classic defence triad denial, repression, and regression. All these defences may be useful, if employed from time to time, to give a child temporary respite from otherwise overwhelming anxiety. If, however, any one of them becomes immutable, personality difficulties or repudiation of treatment may result.[12,55,60,61]

Honest acknowledgement of a child's disability, and encouragement to talk about it, coupled with obvious pleasure in, and reminders concerning, his intact faculties, may be of more value.[77] If a child can see his illness as only a relative handicap, this will help.[78] A child should be constantly challenged with attainable goals. In this way 'his functional disability will remain relative, and not become unbearably absolute'.[79]

Some children transcend their illness fears because of their absolute trust in those who care for them.[12,58] Loving, supportive parent-child relationships are crucial in this respect. Where parents can remain hopeful and emotionally close, empathising with, and supporting their child through his experience, less emotional damage will be done. Indeed, where a sick child is certain that he is loved despite his infirmity, and the burden it imposes, an enrichment of emotional life may result.

Finally, it is important to note that even very young children can adjust to illness and treatment despite crippling anxiety, because of their trust in God.[12] The illness or treatment is then viewed as a challenge, part of God's plan for the child. Frequently, but not always, such an attitude mirrors that of the parents. One must always respect any such sustaining philosophy. Similarly, it is always wrong to shatter a child's own instinctive defences. Instead, with care, a relationship can be established in which the child can communicate his exact fears to a sympathetic adult. Reasurrance can then be given, and it is possible to reassure even a very sick child. With our increasingly sophisticated community resources, basic fears such as the fear of loneliness, pain, disfigurement, and unacceptability, can, and should, be vanquished.

## References

1. Ferguson, B. F., 'Preparing Young Children for Hospitalization. A Comparison of Two Methods', *Pediatrics*, **64** (1979), pp. 656–64.
2. Pearson, G. H. J., 'Effect of Operative Procedures on the Emotional Life of the Child', *American Journal of Diseases of Children,* **62** (1941), p. 716.
3. Levy, D. M., 'Psychic Trauma of Operations in Children and a Note on Combat Neurosis', *American Journal of Diseases of Children*, **69** (1945), pp. 7–25.
4. Miller, M. L., 'The Trauma Effect of Surgical Operations in Childhood on the Integrative Functions of the Ego', *Psychoanalysis Quarterly*, **20** (1951), p. 77.
5. Freud, A., 'The Role of Bodily Illness in the Mental Life of Children', *Psychoanalytical Studies of Children*, **7** (1952), p. 69.
6. Blom, G. E., 'The Reactions of Hospitalised Children to Illness', *Pediatrics*, **22** (1958), p. 590.
7. Calef, V., 'Psychological Consequences of Physical Illness in Childhood', *Journal of the American Psychiatric Association*, **7** (1959).
8. Andersson, L. and Hagwall, L., 'Emotional Disturbances in the Burnt Child and his Family', *Lakartidningen*, 74/35 (1977), pp. 2912–15.
9. Schoelly, M. L. and Fraser, A., 'Emotional Reactions in Muscular Dystrophy', *American Journal of Physical Medicine*, **34** (1955), pp. 119–23.
10. Sherwin, A. C. and McCully, R. S., 'Reactions Observed in Boys of Various Ages (Ten to Fourteen) to a Crippling, Progressive, and Fatal Illness (Muscular Dystrophy)', *Journal of Chronic Disease*, (1961), pp. 59–68.
11. Yudkin, S. 'Children and Death', *Lancet*, (1967), p. 37.
12. Burton, L., *The Family Life of Sick Children* (Routledge and Kegan Paul, London, 1975).
13. Burstein, S. and Meichenbaum, D., 'The Work of Worrying in Children Undergoing Surgery', *Abnormal Child Psychology*, 7(2) (1979), pp. 121–32.
14. Sturner, R. A., Rothbaum, F., Visintainer, M. and Wolfer, J., 'The Effects of Stress on Children's Human Figure Drawing', *Journal of Clinical Psychology*, 36 (1980), pp. 324–31.
15. Waechter, E. H., 'Death Anxiety in Children with Fatal Illness' Unpublished doctoral dissertation, Stanford University (1968).
16. Burton, L., 'Tolerating the Intolerable, the Problems Facing Parents and Children Following Diagnosis' in L. Burton (ed.) *Care of the Child Facing Death* (Routledge and Kegan Paul, London, 1974), pp. 16–38.
17. Anderson, E. M. and Spain, B., *The Child with Spina Bifida* (Methuen and Co. Ltd, London, 1977).
18. Green, M., 'Care of the Child with a Long Term Life Threatening Illness', *Pediatrics*, **39** (1967), pp. 441–5.
19. Burton, L., *Vulnerable Children* (Routledge and Kegan Paul, London, 1968).

20. Spence, J. C., 'The Care of Children in Hospital', *British Medical Journal* (1947), p. 125.

21. Bierman, H. R., 'Parent Participation Program in Pediatric Oncology. A Preliminary Report', *Journal of Chronic Disease*, 3 (1956), p. 632.

22. Knudson, A. G. Jnr, and Natterson, J. M., 'Participation of Parents in the Hospital Care of Fatally Ill Children', *Pediatrics*, 26 (1960), p. 482.

23. Steffen, H. and Kelly, P. K., 'Particular Aspects of the Treatment and Rehabilitation of Chronic Cancer Ill Children and Adolescents with Their Families', *Commission of the European Communities Report*, Brussels 1980.

24. Friedman, S. B., Chodoff, P., Mason, J. W. and Hamburg, D. A., 'Behavioural Observations on Parents Anticipating the Death of a Child', *Pediatrics*, (1963), pp. 600–25.

25. Chodoff, P., Stanford, B., Friedman, B. and Hamburg, D. A., 'Stress, Defenses, and Coping Behaviour. Observations in Parents of Children with Malignant Disease', *American Journal of Psychiatry*, 120 (1964), pp. 743–9.

26. Vernick, J. and Karon, M., 'Who's Afraid of Death on a Leukemia Ward?' *American Journal of Diseases of Children*, 109 (1965), pp. 393–7.

27. Saunders, C., 'The Management of Fatal Illness in Childhood', *Proceedings of the Royal Society of Medicine*, 62 (1969), p. 550.

28. Sigler, A. T., 'The Leukemic Child and his Family', in M. Debuskey (ed.) *The Chronically Ill Child and his Family* (Charles Thomas, Illinois, 1970), pp. 53–60.

29. Bozemann, M. F. C., Orbach, E. and Sutherland, A. M., 'The Adaptation of Mothers to the Threatened Loss of Their Children Through Leukemia', *Cancer*, 8 (1955), pp. 1–19.

30. Solnit, A. J. and Green, M., 'Pediatric Management of the Dying Child II. A Study of the Child's Reaction to the Fear of Dying' in A. J. Solnit and S. A. Provence (eds) *Modern Perspectives in Child Development* (International Universities Press, New York, 1963), p. 217.

31. Easson, W. M., 'Care of the Young Patient Who is dying', *Journal of the American Medical Association*, 205 (1968), pp. 63–7.

32. Pill, R., 'The Sociological Aspects of the Case Study Sample' in M. Stacey and Others (eds) *Hospitals, Children and their Families* (Routledge and Kegan Paul, London, 1970).

33. Rutter, M., 'Separation Experience. A New Look at an Old Topic', *Journal of Pediatrics*, 95 (1979), pp. 147–54.

34. Robertson, J., *A Two Year Old Goes to Hospital* (Film) (Tavistock Clinic, London, University Film Library, New York, 1952).

35. Bowlby, J., *Attachment and Loss* (Pelican, London, 1971).

36. Stacey, M., Dearden, R., Pill, R. and Robinson, D., *Hospitals, Children and Their Families* (Routledge and Kegan Paul, London, 1970).

37. Smith, L., 'Effects of Brief Separation from Parent on Young Children', *Journal of Child Psychology*, 16 (1975), pp. 245–54.

38. Bawkin, H., 'Lonliness in Infants', *American Journal of Diseases*, 63, p. 30.

39. Spitz, R. A., 'Hospitalism: an Inquiry into the Genesis of Psychiatric Conditions in Early Childhood', *Psychoanalytical Study of Children*, 1 (1945), p. 53.

40. Prugh, D. G., 'A Study of Emotional Reactions of Children and Families to Hospitalization and Illness', *American Journal of Orthopsy*, 23 (1953), p. 70.

41. Robertson, J., *Young Children in Hospital* (Tavistock, London, 1970).

42. Vermillion, B. D., Ballentine, V. N. and Grosfeld, J. L., 'The Effective Use of a Parent Care Unit for Infants on Surgical Service', *Journal of Pediatric Surgery*, 14 (1979), pp. 321–4.

43. Debuskey, M., 'Orchestration of Care' in M. Debuskey (ed.) *Chronically Ill*

*Child and his Family* (Charles Thomas, Illinois, 1970), pp. 4–21.

44. Oswin, M., *The Empty Hours* (Allen Lane, London, 1971).

45. Oswin, M., 'The Role of Education in Helping the Child with a Potentially Fatal Disease' in L. Burton (ed.) *Care of the Child Facing Death* (Routledge and Kegan Paul, London, 1974).

46. Jensen, R. A. and Comly, H. H., 'Child Parent Problems and the Hospital', *Nerv. Child*, **7** (1948), p. 200.

47. Edwards, C., 'C.F. and the Medical Social Worker', *CF News*, Nov. 1966.

48. Peck, B., 'Effects of Childhood Cancer on Long Term Survivors and Their Families', *British Medical Journal*, (1979), pp. 1327–9.

49. McCollum, A. T. and Gibson, L. E., 'Family Adaptation to the Child with Cystic Fibrosis', *Journal of Pediatrics*, **77** (1970), pp. 571–8.

50. Spock, A. and Stedman, D. J., 'Psychologic Characteristics of Children with Cystic Fibrosis', *North Carolina Medical Journal* (1966), pp. 426–8.

51. Tropauer, A., Franz, M. N. and Dilgard, V., 'Psychological Aspects of the Care of Children with Cystic Fibrosis', *American Journal of Diseases of Children*, **119** (1970), pp. 424–32.

52. Burton, L., 'Some Psychological Considerations Implicit in the Treatment of Pediatric Malignancy', *Proceedings of the Annual Conference of the Canadian Association of Radiologists*, Toronto, 1972.

53. Bergmann, T., (in collaboration with Anna Freud) *Children in Hospital* (International Universities Press, New York, 1965).

54. Schowalter, J. E., 'Psychological Reactions to Physical Illness and Hospitalization in Adolescence', *J. Am. Acad. Child. Psychiat.*, **16** (1977), pp. 500–16.

55. Chodoff, P., 'Adjustment to Disability. Some Observations on Patients with M.S', *Journal of Chronic Diseases*, (1959), p. 653.

56. Mead, J., *Helen's Victory* (Health Horizon, London, 1969).

57. Burton, L., 'Cancer Children', *New Society*, **455** (1971), pp. 1040–3.

58. Morrisey, J. R., 'Children's Adaptation to Fatal Illness', *Social Work*, (1963), pp. 81–8.

59. Green, M., 'Care of the Dying Child', *Pediatrics*, **40** (1967), pp. 492–8.

60. Lawler, R. H., Nakielny, W. and Wright, N., 'Psychological Implications of Cystic Fibrosis', *Canadian Medical Association Journal*, **94** (1966), pp. 1043–6.

61. Bruch, Hilde and Hewlett, Irma, 'Psychologic Aspects of the Medical Management of Diabetes in Children', *Psychosomatic Medicine*, **9** (1947), pp. 205–9.

62. Pinkerton, P., 'Managing the Psychological Aspects of CF', *Arizona Medicine*, **26** (1969), pp. 345–51.

63. Lansky, S. and Gendel, M., 'Symbiotic Regressive Behaviour Patterns in Childhood Malignancy. A Pattern Characterized by a Severe Separation Anxiety in the Sick Child and a Parent, and Extreme Social Withdrawal of the Pair', *Clinical Pediatrics*, **17** (1978), pp. 133–8.

64. Green, M. and Solnit, A. J. Solnit, 'Reactions to the Threatened Loss of a Child: A Vulnerable Child Syndrome', *Pediatrics*, (1964), pp. 58–66.

65. Falkman, C., 'C.F. A Psychological Study of 52 Children and Their Families', *Acta Paediatrica Scandinavica Suppl.*, **269** (1979), pp. 1–93.

66. Dorner, S., 'The Relationship of Physical Handicap to Stress in Families with an Adolescent with Spina Bifida', *Developmental Medicine and Child Neurology*, **17** (1975), pp. 765–76.

67. Wallis, H., 'Stress Reactions in Children', *Therapiewoche*, **29** (1979), pp. 4942–7.

68. Chabon, S. S. and Chabon, R. S., 'Annotated Bibliography of Health Care Books for Children', *American Journal of Diseases of Children*, **133**(2) (1979), pp. 184–6.

69. Powazek, M., Goff, J. R., Schyving, J. and Paulson, M. A., 'Emotional Reactions of Children to Isolation in a Cancer Hospital', *Journal of Pediatrics*, **92** (1978), pp. 834–7.

70. Pidgeon, V. A., 'Child Thought and Counselling Implications in the Hospital', *Patient Counselling and Health Education*, **1** (1978), pp. 4–7.

71. Henley, T. F. and Albam, B., 'A Psychiatric Study of Muscular Dystrophy. The Role of the Social Worker', *American Journal of Physical Medicine*, **34** (1955), pp. 258–64.

72. Rosenstein, B. J., 'Cystic Fibrosis of the Pancreas. Impact on Family Functioning' in M. Debuskey (ed.) *The Chronically Ill Child and His Family* (Charles Thomas, Illinois, 1970), pp. 23–33.

73. Lewis, M., 'The Management of Parents of Acutely Ill Children in the Hospital', *American Journal of Orthopsy*, **32** (1962), pp. 60–6.

74. Tonyan, A. B., 'Role of the Nurse in a Children's Cancer Clinic', *Pediatrics*, **40** (1967), pp. 532.

75. Jessner, L. and Kaplan, S., 'Observations on the Emotional Reaction of Children to Tonsillectomy and Adenoidectomy' in M. J. E. Senn (ed.) *Problems in Infancy and Childhood* (New York, 1948).

76. Goldberg, R. T., Isralsky, M. and Shwachman, H., 'Vocational Development and Adjustment of Adolescents with CF', *Archives of Physical and Medical Rehabilitation*, **60** (1979), pp. 369–74.

77. Rieder, T. and Wagner, K. D., 'Reaction Types and the Experience of Disease', *Kinderarztl Prax.*, **43** (1975), pp. 49–53.

78. Hvizdalla, E. V., Miace, T. D. and Barnard, P. J., 'A Summer Camp for Children with Cancer', *Medical Pediatric Oncology*, **4** (1978), pp. 71–5.

79. Haller, J. A., 'A Healthy Attitude to Chronic Illness' in M. Debusky (ed.) *The Chronically Ill Child and His Family* (Charles Thomas, Springfield, Illinois, 1970).

# 11 PSYCHOLOGICAL TREATMENT OF CHILDHOOD NEUROSES

Martin Herbert

This chapter focuses on some of the more general theoretical and practical issues which relate to the psychological treatment of neurotic disorders of childhood. Although the author trained as a child psychotherapist (play therapist) he now makes use of behavioural methods (within an eclectic framework) in his work at the *Child Treatment Research Unit* in the Psychology Department at the University of Leicester.

For these reasons a broadly based integrative approach is put forward in this chapter. Various 'schools' of thought are represented in greater detail in other chapters. The reader will be directed to useful supplementary reading.

Our starting point must be with a definition. What are the so-called neurotic problems which beset children? There is a general consensus among clinical and statistical studies confirming the validity of a clinical distinction between those disorders which primarily lead to emotional disturbance or distress for the child himself (e.g. anxiety, shyness, depression, feelings of inferiority and timidity) and those which involve mainly the kinds of antisocial behaviour (e.g. destructiveness, aggression, lying, stealing and disobedience) which disrupt the wellbeing of others, notably those in frequent contact with the child.[1] The former category, the so-called 'neurotic' or 'emotional' disorders, are manifested by about 2.5 per cent of pre-adolescent children; their prevalence increases somewhat by adolescence. Boys and girls are about equally prone to neurotic problems.

The child is a developing being and as such, he manifests many 'symptoms' which are in fact normal and which disappear in time as a function of growing up.[2] For most children emotional and behaviour problems manifest themselves briefly at certain stages of development — perhaps associated with particular 'crises' of development[3] — and then become minimal or disappear completely. Prospective studies indicate that among the problems which decline in frequency with age are elimination (toilet training) problems, speech problems, fears and thumb sucking. Problems such as insufficient appetite and lying reach a peak early and then subside. Many problems show high frequencies round about or just before school-starting age, then decline in prevalence, and later rise again at puberty. Among these are restless sleep, disturbing dreams, physical timidity, irritability, attention-demanding, over-dependence, sombreness, jealously and, in boys, food-finickiness. Among the problems which show little or no relationship to age is oversensitiveness. The high 'spontaneous remission' rate of many childhood disorders must be taken into account in evaluating the success of different treatment methods.[4]

We know as a result of longitudinal studies that for the most part, children who suffer from emotional disorders become reasonably well-adjusted adults; they are almost as likely to grow up 'normal' as children drawn at random from the general population.[5] You could say that these difficulties are the emotional equivalent of 'growing pains'. But that is not to deny that they sometimes endure and reach levels of intensity which cause everybody concerned with the youngster, and not least, the child, great distress. Clinicians tend to designate these problems as *neuroses* or *neurotic disorders*.

The term neurosis seems to be used broadly at times, as a short-hand term for something as pervasive as emotional disturbance: it can be applied to a set of attitudes;[6] and it can also be defined narrowly and technically.[7,8] The neurotic child — whatever the usage — is invariably a suffering individual. What separates behaviours defined as 'neurotic' from the anxiety, avoidances, fears, indecisiveness and obsessions shown by all children at one time or another, is the frequency (rate), intensity and persistence (duration) with which they are manifested, and the sheer number of problems with which they are associated (see Figure 11.1, No. 3).

The generic term neurosis can encompass:

(a)  Feelings of unhappiness, distress, misery;

(b)  Vague feelings that life is not being lived as meaningfully, effectively, joyfully as it should be;

(c)  A feeling of having lost control;

(d)  A loss of the ability to make decisions;

(e)  A loss of the ability to make choices;

(f)  A loss of the feeling of being real, vital, committed to, enthusiastic about, life;

# Figure 11.1: Assessment Framework

**5 Antecedent events**
- 3 a Distal antecedents
- b Proximal antecedents

**2 Setting events**
- Persons
- Places
- Times
- Situations

**1 BEHAVIOUR (target problems)**

**3 Parameters**
- Frequency
- Intensity
- Number
- Duration
- Sense/meaning

**7 Diagnostic implications**
- Personal (emotional)
- Social
- Ongoing development
- Learning
- Others

**8.**
- Attitudes toward the self
- Integration
- Reality-orientation
- Autonomy
- Perception of reality
- Growth, development and self-actualisation
- Environmental mastery

**6 Consequent events**
- a Proximal outcomes
- b Distal outcomes

**4 Organismic variables**
- Age
- Sex
- Congenital-genetic factors
- Brain functioning
- Personality and arousal
- Health and physical impairment
- Temperament
- Autonomic reactivity
- Stress proneness
- Cognition — IQ
- Achievement level

Source: Adapted from Herbert.30

(g) A sense of conflict, apathy, aimlessness;

(h) A sense of alienation (with self and/or society);

(i) A sense of being compelled to do things against one's will;

(j) An avoidance of situations/people/objects one shouldn't have to avoid;

(k) A sense of restriction, narrowing of one's horizons because of vague apprehensions or acute fear;

(l) A sense of emotional turmoil (anger, fear, anxiety, dread, guilt, depression, disgust);

(m) A feeling of helplessness, of not being fully in control of one's life;

(n) Physical ailments/malaise which have no organic basis.

Ultimately, the clinical judgement of a child's psychosocial or mental status is made in individual terms, taking into account his particular circumstances. It involves an estimate of the consequences that flow from the client's specific thoughts, feelings and behaviours and general life-style, with particular reference to his personal and emotional well-being, his social relationships, his ongoing development and self-actualisation, his ability to work effectively and (in the case of children) to learn academically, and his accessibility to socialisation. All are subject to disruption in neurotic disorders, and are gravely affected in the conduct disorders of childhood and adolescence; they figure consequently among the goals or objectives set in treatment programmes. Other factors to be considered are the child's self-esteem and competence (see Figure 11.1, No. 8).

There is no general agreement about the defining attributes of psychopathology or, on the opposite side of the coin, positive mental health. Jahoda[9] provides an interesting discussion of these important issues. The criteria she lists as significant are included in the framework for assessment provided above (see column 8, Figure 11.1).

## Models of Intervention

It is common for the two clusters of problems described earlier to be thought of as either over-controlled (internalised) or under-controlled (externalised) patterns of behaviour. These 'directional metaphors' are illuminating, but also misleading if applied too rigidly or literally to individual cases.

As we shall see, they contain theoretical assumptions. Thus 'acting out' behaviour (e.g. aggressive, delinquent actions) may be seen as the outward and visible signs of inner turmoil and conflict. Behaviour therapists may reject such interpretations and deal directly with the presenting problems. On the other hand the therapist using insight therapy with children and adolescents engages in procedures which will give the patient insight into the unconscious meaning of his aggressive symptoms, and into the relationship between his motivations and his behaviour. It is assumed that this insight will give him greater control over his behaviour. Many of our motives are unconscious and according to this perspective, it is impossible to come to terms with an 'invisible enemy'. The therapist tries to make the invisible visible, the unconscious conscious, so that reality can be grappled with.

## Insight-based Therapies

It would be safe to say that insight therapies tend to be 'talking' therapies, although action therapies like behaviour modification *can* generate 'insights'. The patient or client does a lot of talking about himself, his life, his early history, his personal relationships, his work, ambitions, fears and worries. The psychotherapist, to a great or lesser extent, also talks — offering interpretations of the patient's conflicts and problems, reassurance and sometimes advice. He tries to direct the person's thoughts and actions into potentially fruitful channels. Psychotherapy, because of all this soul-searching, has been described by some people as the confessional of secular people. Confession undoubtedly does have a therapeutic effect for anxiety and guilt-ridden people. If the child is very young and therefore unreflexive, conventional psychotherapy is inappropiate.

## Psychoanalytic and Neo-psychoanalytic Perspectives

Sigmund Freud, the founder of psychoanalysis, was an exponent of verstehende or 'understanding' psychology. The classical Freudian theory is primarily a doctrine about mental energy (psychic energy). There is a metaphor in Freud's exposition, in which the person is like an energy system: a hydraulic system in which energy flows, gets diverted, overflows, or becomes dammed-up. In all children (it is postulated), there is a limited amount of energy, and if it gets discharged in one way, there is that much less energy to be discharged in another way. This mental energy serves to determine the psychosexual stages — oral, anal and phallic — through which the child's mind and personality develop and become partitioned. The structural aspects of personality — ego, id, superego — were introduced by Freud in an attempt to deal with the central problem of psychological conflict; the theme of 'the person divided against himself/herself'.

The mind, Freud theorised, is cut across by a critically important barrier, separating the unconscious from the conscious elements, the atavistic from the social/moral. The id contains the blind striving of both the life and death instincts and is the source of all our motives, drives and energies. The ego is the rational section of the personality, and the superego is the moral and ethical part of the child's being, akin to conscience. The ego has at its command several 'defence mechanisms' — repression, rationalisation, fantasy, sublimation and regression — with which to control the balance and distribution of energy. If this control has not been satisfactorily achieved in the past, the repression barrier, which has kept the unconscious impulses of the mind at bay, may break down under stress or frustration.

As a result, the unconscious elements may then come to the surface to the accompaniment of anxiety, and in the compromise form of neurotic symptoms, producing (in the child) internalised neurotic problems or (alternatively) 'acting-out' conduct disorders.[10] Psychoanalysis, with its concentration on instincts, is a motivationally based theory which assumes determinism in all human behaviour, the existence and significant influence of unconscious mental processes, and the perennial nature of psychological conflict and anxiety in both normal personality development and in the evolution of psychopathology.

Freud treated no childen directly, although his report in 1937 on 'Little Hans', a child analysed vicariously, proved highly influential.[11] His views of childhood and its aberrations were based largely upon reconstructions of the early years derived from the free associations, dreams and memories of adult neurotic patients. Freud went on to say that abnormal mental phenomena are simply exaggerations of normal phenomena, and that a patient's symptoms represent, in essence, the outcome of his attempts to meet his problems as best he can; in this way he bridged the gap between normal and abnormal behaviour.

The practical implications of the psychoanalytic or neo-psycho-analytic approaches to childhood problems — the latter best illustrated by the work of Anna, Freud's daughter[12] — is that treatment usually takes the classical one-to-one (so-called 'dyadic') approach in which the therapist works directly with the child. Classical Freudian psychoanalysis has, over the years become elaborated, transformed, and in the hands of some of its cross-disciplinary practitioners, diluted — it is called the psychodynamic approach. Whatever it is called, the *conventional* methods of psychoanalytic psychotherapy used with adults are not always suited to the needs and capacities of children. Children are not notably introspective when younger. Being unskilled in this way, they are not always able to put their anxieties into words. Additionally, youngsters are not always able, willing or interested, to explore their past life. They are too close to the episodes that are thought by psychoanalysts to be crucial in the development of neuroses, to enjoy talking about them; they will not or cannot always free-associate. The main problem is that the incentive to participate in analysis is missing because children do not necessarily conceptualise themselves as being or having problems; indeed they are often brought for treatment against their will.

## Play Therapy

A special kind of therapy ('play therapy') is available which makes use of the child's familiar and natural mode of expression — play — and this provides a background for the therapist to discuss and interpret problems with the youngster. Theories of the importance of play in childhood go a long way back. As early as the 18th century, Rousseau advocated the study of children's play in order to understand and educate them. There have been several theories put forward to explain the meaning and utility of play in childhood;*

---

*Erik Erikson, in his classic book *Childhood and Society*[3] states that 'modern play therapy is based on the observation that a child made insecure by a secret hate against or fear of the natural protectors of his play in family and neighbourhood seems able to use the protective sanctions of an understanding adult to regain some play peace . . . today this role is the play therapist's.' (p. 215).

they generally emphasise its function as a means of preparation for life, as a natural process of learning and as a means of catharsis — release from tensions and of excess physical energies. In many ways play, for children, is life itself; they develop their personalities and their abilities to get on with other children, while indulging in it.

Anna Freud used children's play in a manner analogous to the use of dreams with adults; she analysed play so as to uncover unconscious conflicts. This involved the interpretation of the symbolic meanings, the unconscious motives, underlying drawings, paintings, games and other forms of imaginitive play. She transposed classical psychoanalytic theory into a system of child analysis.

Over the years there have been several offshoots of psychoanalytical play therapy and also systems of play therapy which are not in this mould at all. (Melanie Klein and Margaret Lowenfeld have been eminent innovators.) The active forms of play therapy have much in common with the desensitisation techniques used in behaviour therapy. Other forms of play therapy — relationship therapy and nondirective therapy — have evolved and continue to be used.

Virginia Mae Axline[13] describes the nondirective form of play therapy. This is based on the assumption that the individual has within himself, not only the ability to solve his own problems satisfactorily, but also a growth impulse that makes mature behaviour more satisfying than immature behaviour. Axline makes the point that the approach is based upon the fact that play is the child's natural medium of self-expression. An opportunity is given to children to 'play out' their feelings and problems just as, in certain types of adult therapy, individuals 'talk out' their difficulties. (See Axline[14] for a fascinating example of a child Dibs' treatment from this perspective.)

The basic principles which guide the therapist are as follows:

1. The therapist develops a warm friendly relationship with the child.
2. She accepts the child exactly as he is.
3. She establishes a feeling of permissiveness in the relationship so that the child feels entirely free to express his feelings.
4. The therapist is alert to recognise the feelings expressed by the child and to reflect those feeling back to him in such a manner that he gains insight into his behaviour.

5. She maintains a deep respect for the child's ability to solve his own problems if given an opportunity to do so. The responsibility for making choices and for instituting change is the child's.
6. The clinician does not attempt to hurry therapy along. It is a gradual process.
7. She does not attempt to direct the child's actions or conversation in any manner. The child leads the way and the therapist follows.
8. The therapist establishes only those limitations to the child's behaviour that are necessary to anchor the therapy to the world of reality and to make the child aware of his responsibility in the relationship.

Put at its simplest, child psychotherapy — whatever modality it takes — involves the modification or reshaping of attitudes and feelings. The therapist does not simply discuss personal and situational events with the child or attempt to explain the inappropriateness of his behaviour or the self-defeating attitudes towards himself and his environment. The youngster is helped indirectly to see for himself that what he is doing and feeling is unadaptive. The child may need an opportunity to express (i.e. *ventilate*) those feelings which he has suppressed or displaced onto some convenient scapegoat. His attitudes and defences need careful analysis over a broad front.

## The Analysis of 'Defensive/coping' Styles

From a very young age, individuals discover and utilise complex 'defensive' reactions[10] designed to protect and enhance the gradually evolving self-image. All human beings old enough to have acquired even a rudimentary self-image seem to need, and indeed strive to perceive themselves in a favourable light. A reasonable agreement between the self-concept ('myself as I am') and the concept of the ideal self ('myself as I would like to be') is one of the most important conditions for personal happiness and for satisfaction in life. Marked discrepancies arouse anxiety, and are associated with psychological problems.[5] Such discrepancies are a feature of neurotic personalities. Because the self is the central integrating aspect of the person any threat to its valuation can be a threat to the very being of the individual. The defensive strategies and tactics such as rationalisation, denial, over-compensation, fantasy and displacement, soften anxieties and failures and guard the integrity of the ego by increasing the feeling of personal work. When used to excess, involving as they do a degree of self-deception, they may be thought of as neurotic. They would form the basis (in part) of a therapeutic or counselling discussion, particularly with the older youth.

Self-esteem is central to certain features of the neuroses or what might be termed neurotic attitudes. Coopersmith[15] conducted a series of studies of self-esteem applying the techniques of clinical, laboratory and field investigation. The subjects consisted of a representative sample of normal boys aged ten to twelve, who were followed from their pre-adolescent stage to early adulthood. Various indices of self-esteem were used. Coopersmith provides evidence that the optimum conditions required for the achievement of high self-esteem in children are a combination of firm enforcement of limits on the child's behaviour together with a marked degree of freedom (autonomy) within these limits. As long as the parentally imposed constraints are backed up by social norms outside the home, this provides the youngster with a clear idea of an orderly and trustworthy social reality which, in turn, gives him a solid basis for his own actions. Coopersmith found that children with low self-esteem (associated with laissez-faire parenting) presented a picture of discouragement and depression. They tended to feel isolated, unlovable, incapable of expressing or defining themselves and too weak to confront or overcome their deficiencies. They were anxious about angering others and shrank from exposing themselves to the limelight in any way.

Such a finding suggests that rather than concentrating almost entirely on self-understanding, attitudes and feelings, professional efforts may have to be directed to the situations of parents, family, peer-group, school and work place which form, or at least sustain, the psychological conditions of children. It may be unrealistic to expect weekly interviews with therapists or weekly counselling sessions in groups, to have critical effects, when situational conditions are neglected.

**The Systems (Ecological) Orientation: Family Therapy**

Systems theorists are agreed in focusing not so much on the

allegedly 'problematic' child but on the nexus of relationships within which he functions.

Family therapy involves a basic redefinition of the therapeutic task. There is an attempt to conceptualise the client as part of a complex network of interacting social systems any aspects of which may have a bearing on his present predicament. Family therapy involves a broad view of what constitutes a 'case'. Whereas the early child guidance treatment model tended to identify the nominated patient as the unit of attention (for example the child; with lip service paid to the family as his background) diagnostic thinking has lately been influenced greatly by interactional frames of reference (explicit in systems thinking). Thus the unit of attention, particularly in relation to the family, is far more broadly conceived, and the focus of help not prejudged as the nominated client — the neurotic child. (Family therapy is discussed in Chapter 6.)

The unit of attention is defined as *the family* (or one of its subsystems) rather than the *individual in the context of his family*. Increasing understanding of the effects of group influences on individual behaviour has also modified views of what should be taken into account in assessment and treatment. The search for the specific and crucial conditions in the child's cumulative experience with his family, and other agents of socialisation, is an ancient one. The following couplet with its ironic comment on child care practices is from Aristophanes and dates back to the Fifth Century BC:

Come listen now to the good old days
when children, strange to tell,
Were seen not heard, led a simple life,
in short, were brought up well.

In part, the scientific inquiry into childhood arises out of a conviction about the extensive power and reach of early experience; a belief that optimal care and training of children during the impressionable years of life, will function as a kind of vaccination — innoculating them against the future problems of adolescence and adulthood.

One still hears occasionally what used to be a popular catch-phrase: 'There are no problem children only problem parents'. This statement refers to an explanation of why children become maladjusted, i.e. fail to adapt to society's norms. As such it represents an exaggeration of a partial truth. Provided the enthusiasm to over-simplify explanatory theories is tempered by a realisation that causation of childhood disorders is seldom linear, generally multi-factorial and almost always complex, there *are* hints for problem-remediation to be gleaned from studies of parent-child relations.

Of particular interest is the finding in clinic-attending patients that by comparison with antisocial conduct-disordered youths, the over-inhibited neurotic youngsters were most likely to have been restricted and constrained at home.[16] The mothers of anxious children tended to show infantilising, overprotective attitudes.[17] Unsocialised, aggressive, delinquent youths most often came from families in which parent-child interactions were marked by mutual suspicion, hostility and rejection. The parents punished severely and were inconsistent and unjust. One can speculate that it is difficult for the child to identify with such parents, and thus the aggression they provoke is not directed against the self (intro-punitive) as it is in the case of a child with normal conscience-development. It is turned outward and vented on society.

Factor analytic and computer techniques have been used in order to reduce the rich variety of childhood and parental behaviours to a few main dimensions.[5] For example, Schaefer[18] describes parental attitudes in terms of the interactions of only two main orthogonal attributes. One dimension involves attitudes that are 'warm' (or loving) at one extreme, and 'rejecting' (or hostile) at the other; while the other dimension is made up of attitudes which are restrictive (controlling) at one extreme, and permissive (encouraging autonomy) at the other (Figure 11.2).

Reviews of research[19] into child-rearing techniques suggest an empirical basis for the notion that there is a 'happy medium', that the extremes of permissiveness and restrictiveness both entail risks. A blend of permissiveness and a warm, encouraging and accepting attitude fits the recommendations of child-rearing specialists who are concerned with fostering the sort of children who are socially responsible and outgoing, friendly, competent, creative and reasonably independent and self-assertive (admittedly Western values).

The balance is perhaps best illustrated in the philosophy of what Baumrind[20] calls the 'authoritative parent'. This kind of mother attempts to direct her child's activities in a rational manner determined by the issues involved in particular disciplinary situations. She encourages verbal give-and-take, and shares with the

Figure 11.2: Empirical Relationships Between Parent Variables[18] and Child Behaviours[19]

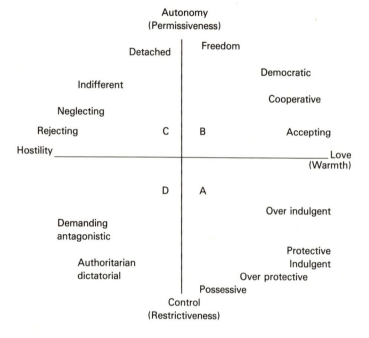

| | Restrictiveness | Permissiveness |
|---|---|---|
| Warmth | Submissive, dependent, polite, neat, obedient<br>Minimal aggression<br>A Maximum rule enforcement (boys)<br>Dependent, not friendly, not creative<br>Maximal compliance | Active, socially outgoing, creative, successfully aggressive<br>Minimal rule enforcement (boys)<br>Facilitates adult role taking<br>B Minimal self-aggression (boys)<br>Independent, friendly, creative, low projective hostility |
| Hostility | 'Neurotic' problems<br>More quarrelling and shyness with peers<br>D Socially withdrawn<br>Low in adult role taking<br>Maximal self-aggression (boys) | Delinquency<br>C Noncompliance<br>Maximal aggression |

children the reasoning behind her policy. She values both the child's self expression and his so-called 'instrumental attributes' (respect for authority, work and the like). Baumrind states that the evidence points to 'a synthesis and balancing of strongly opposing forces of tradition and innovation, divergence and convergence, accommodation and assimilation, cooperation and autonomous expression, tolerance and principled intractability'.

## An Eclectic Approach

Developmental counselling, based upon findings like these, can play a preventative as well as remedial role.[5,21] The provision of information to parents — their realisation that their child's problem is not unique or necessarily 'hopeless' — may release them from worried preoccupation with their offspring's every action, and thereby liberate the youngster from unbearable tension. Thus counselling, 'sympathetic' listening, direct advice or action (e.g. behavioural programming), interpretation and insight-giving, may make up a modern clinic's armamentarium.

However, whatever the theoretical framework of a contemporary clinic, it is fairly common practice for a child to be made to feel at ease in a playroom in which he can paint, construct things on a sand tray with miniatures (e.g. 'world games'), act out dramas with dolls and puppets, be aggressive with guns and knives and, in a secure and trustful ethos, give expression to a wide range of feelings and fantasies. The skilled therapist may detect recurrent themes in the child's play, preoccupations which point to anxieties, conflicts or areas of tension in the family or at school, problems which are impeding his development. The use of projective material or conversation for communication will help the therapist to diagnose and then later to treat the child's problem. The child's problem is so often connected with parental actions and attitudes that the clinic will usually require both parents to come regularly with the child, in some cases as mediators of a behavioural programme but sometimes for personal counselling. Increasingly behavioural work is carried out in the home or school setting.[22]

All therapies enjoy some degree of success;[23] and this begs the question 'Why?' What does this diversity of theoretical and technical approaches have in common, if anything? Some dynamic theorists have come to accept the idea that psychotherapy might best be viewed as a learning process. Dollard and Miller[24] reinterpreted psychoanalytic psychotherapy in learning terms such as reinforcement, generalisation and extinction. A significant aspect of their effort was that they found it necessary to postulate many additional processes, such as mediated discrimination and generalisation, verbal labels and cue-producing responses, and approach-avoidance conflict on the symbolic level, in order to account for the higher mental processes that were involved in the phenomena they were attempting to explain. In addition, they made a number of assumptions about learned social responses in order to account for the social aspects of the patient's difficulties and the transference relationship between the patient and therapist. In making these assumptions about the higher mental processes and social relationships, Dollard and Miller went far beyond the simplistic concepts of learning prevalent at that time, conceptions that were derived largely from the animal laboratory. Franz Alexander[25] emphasised that the most significant learning occurs within the context of the interpersonal relationship of the therapist and the patient.

The particular theoretical explanation of a therapy may not necessarily be valid; there may well be alternative explanations. For example, in dynamic psychotherapy it is claimed that interpretations have important effects. However, an interpretation may be viewed as a complex communication between therapist and child. This communication contains information about the attitudes and motives of the therapist and provides cues that the child may interpret as indicating what is expected of him. The same applies to behaviour therapy. The genuine controlling variables may also be considerably different in reality from those formulated by way of explanation of the behaviour therapist. (See reference 26 for a recent synthesis.)

The evidence presented by Murray and Jacobson[27] strongly suggests that both traditional and behavioural psychotherapy achieve their results as a results as a function of crucial processes for which there is little place in the theoretical system of these therapies. The explanation of traditional therapy in terms of personal growth and personality reorganisation does not take sufficient account of social learning and social influence processes; the explanations of behavioural therapies do not adequately recognise the importance of cognitive and emotional response systems operating within interpersonal relationships (see also reference 28).

## Behaviour Therapy

Behaviour therapy is based upon a social learning model in which abnormal behaviours are viewed as the manner in which the child has learned to cope with the challenge and stress of living in a changing, complex and increasingly more impersonal social environment. In this view, it is not possible to draw clear cut lines of demarcation between those who fall into the diagnostic categories of neurosis or psychiatric disorder and those who do not. We are referring, in most cases, to behavioural continua. A basic assumption of this approach is that psychiatric disorders, by and large, are exaggerations, deficits or handicapping combinations of behaviours common to all children. O'Leary and Wilson[29] state that since abnormal behaviour is learned and maintained in the same way as normal behaviour, it can be treated directly through the application of social learning principles rather than indirectly by 'working through' these underlying problems.

The approach of the Child Treatment Research Unit (based on broadly conceived developmental and social learning theory and the so-called triadic model) has provided encouraging evidence[30] of the ability of parents to help themselves and their problematic children over a wide range of problems. The triadic model recognises the profound influence that parents have on their children's development and mental health. As parents and teachers exert a significant foundational influence during the impressionable years of early childhood, they are usually in a strong position to facilitate prosocial learning and adjustment, and moderate the genesis of behaviour problems. Additionally, they are on hand and therefore in a good position to extend the beneficial changes (brought about in therapy) over time, and to generalise them across various life-situations. If it is accepted that problematic behaviours of childhood occur in part as a function of faulty learning processes, then there is a case for arguing that problems can most effectively be modified *where they occur*, by making good the deficits or by changing the social training of the child, and the contingencies supplied by social agents.

## Identifying Controlling Variables (Figure 11.1 nos. 4, 5 and 6)

Kazdin[31] observes, in his history of behaviour therapy, that the discipline has grown and diversified out of all recognition since its formal beginnings in the late 1950s and early 1960s. It is no longer the monolithic entity it once was; behaviour therapy has become so diverse in its conceptualisations of behaviour, research methods, and techniques, that no unifying scheme or set of assumptions can incorporate all extant techniques. He states that although behaviour therapy emphasises the principles of classical and operant conditioning it is not restricted to them; it draws upon principles from other branches of experimental psychology such as social and developmental psychology. The importance of 'private events' or the cognitive mediation of behaviour is recognised; and a major role is attributed to vicarious and symbolic learning processes, for example, modelling. Thus, when behaviour therapists set out to identify controlling variables, two categories of controlling variable are generally considered: current environmental variables (antecedent and consequent events nos. 5/6, Figure 11.1) and organismic variables (no. 4 Figure 11.1).[30] The behavioural assessment is based on the concept of a functional relationship with the environment and vice versa. The contemporary causes of problem behaviour may exist in the client's environment or in his own thoughts, feelings or bodily processes (organismic variables) and they may exert their influence in several ways: as eliciting or discriminative antecedent stimuli or as outcomes (consequences) of a reinforcing kind. The development of inappropriate strategies (or the failure to acquire appropriate strategies) for coping with life tasks, might be due to faulty training and/or modelling or other environmental deficiencies. They might be a consequence of neurological defects or other inherited or acquired impairments. Excellent accounts of the experimental derivations of these ideas are to be found in Bandura[32,33] and Rimm and Masters.[34]

Organismic variables include individual differences produced by age, sex, genetic constitution, physiology and by past learning. There is evidence, for example, that some children — from birth — are difficult: they are more likely to be sickly, or to have feeding and sleeping problems. Being more difficult to rear, they make extra demands that the parents are at times unable to meet.[5] The child's condition acts on the parents' feelings of inadequacy, and so the child, unwittingly, contributes to his own problems. Although difficult children are likely to develop emotional or behavioural problems, they do not always do so. About 30 per cent (and the difficult ones are a small minority) adjust slowly but well. The baby born with a hypersensitive, tense and anxious outlook may, through affectionate and strength-giving parents, emerge as a healthy child; that is, a strong environment may develop a child's limited potential.

Behaviour therapists find it useful to distinguish the historical (distal antecedents) and the contemporary causes (proximal antecedents) of problem behaviour. Most people working in the behaviour therapy field adopt an interactional position — the view that behaviour results from an interaction between the current situation and individual differences (biological and psychosocial).

Some critics, sceptical about the theoretical underpinning of behaviour therapy, consider behavioural treatment simply as a technology. Certainly, the techniques can be utilised and researched *without* commitment to any distinctive foundational theory. However, others disagree[28] with an atheoretical perspective. Kazdin[31] points out in a recent review that the last 15 years or so have seen major advances in the behavioural treatment of children's problems. There is a wide range of empirically based therapeutic procedures from which to choose in planning an intervention.

## Behavioural Treatment

For reasons given at the beginning of the chapter, only a few brief examples of methods will be given in this section.

### Treatment of Neurotic (i.e. Phobic) Anxiety by Systematic Desensitisation

Unadaptive (phobic) anxiety is formulated by behaviour therapists as a learned reaction, which is elicited in situations in which it is not objectively called for, in that no real danger exists. The dangers are often in the mind of the child, in the form of anticipated consequences of a dreadful kind, or other negative evaluations of the situation. Diagnosis is difficult because of the prevalence of children's fears which 'look' unreasonable from an adult point of view.

The procedure called systematic desensitisation involves the presentation of the anxiety-provoking stimulus while preventing the anxiety response from occurring. This is achieved by training the child to engage in an activity that is incompatible with the anxiety reaction. The stimulus may be *imaginal* (conjured up by the child's fantasy in imagination) or presented *in vivo* (the child being exposed to the real-life stimulus).

There can be little doubt that as a package, systematic desensitisation works, both in the short and longer term,[30,35] producing success rates of between 70 and 90 per cent, which represent substantially better than spontaneous remission rates. The success of desensitisation goes beyond fears and phobias related to social situations, death, injury, illness, animals and sexual encounters. There is, however, a lot of doubt that we know *how* it works, despite the many explanations offered; the only necessary condition for change seems to be exposure to the feared object or situation. For children, participant modelling by the therapist is a helpful ingredient. The essential role of muscular relaxation and the presentation of hierarchies of anxiety-provoking stimuli — especially with children — has been brought into question. In general, longer durations of exposure to phobic stimuli result in greater fear reduction, irrespective of type of fear.

### Treatment of Stress Disorders by Problem-Solving

The rationale for these methods is formulated as follows:[36]

> Much of what we view clinically as 'abnormal behaviour' or 'emotional disturbance' may be viewed as ineffective behaviour and its consequences, in which the individual is unable to resolve certain situational problems in his life and his inadequate attempts to do so are having undesirable effects, such as anxiety, depression, and the creation of additional problems. (p. 107)

Youngsters can be taught rational thinking, stress-inoculation techniques and problem-solving strategies.[30] The aim of training children in problem-solving skills is to provide them with a general coping strategy for a variety of difficult situations. The method has been used to help children and adolescents to deal more effectively with a variety of conflict situations (e.g. arriving at mutually acceptable decisions with parents, developing cooperation with the peer group). Its prime advantage as a training method is the provision of principles so that the person can function as his own 'therapist'. It is a variant of self-control training, directed towards the objective of encouraging the youngster to think and work things out for himself.

Whereas the nature of the cognitive problems associated with adult anxiety and depression — to take two examples — can be conceptualised as *cognitive errors*, the cognitive problems and the focus of treatment in child cognitive-behavioural therapy are most often *cognitive absences*. Kendall[37] explains that the child fails to engage in the cognitive, information-processing activities of an active problem-solver and refrains from initiating the reflective thought processes that can control behaviour. Indeed he may lack the cognitive skills needed to carry out crucial abstract, analytical mental activities.

### Treatment of Dysfunctional Emotion by Developing Cognitive Self-management Skills

Stress-inoculation training has been used successfully[38] in the self-management of phobic anxiety, anger and pain. Children are provided with a prospective set of skills and defences so as to deal with future crises. The training programme has three phases: (a) the first, educational in nature, provides the child with a conceptual framework for understanding the nature of his problem; (b) a number of behavioural and cognitive coping skills arising from the conceptual framework, are rehearsed by the child; and (c) the opportunity is provided for the child to practise his coping skills while being exposed to a variety of real stresses and/or practice by means of imagery and behavioural rehearsal.

## Review of Outcome Studies

When we ask how effective child therapy is, we inevitably beg several further questions; effective for whom?; to what purpose?; in what context?; for how long? The *outcome* of therapy is not a unitary variable; it differs according to the perspective of the child, relatives, therapist, peers and others. Critics suggest that psycho-dynamic approaches to children's problems do not improve on the rate at which they would get better without treatment (i.e. the so-called 'spontaneous remission' rate). These views have not gone unchallenged. A major problem is the paucity of hard evidence about the effectiveness of treatment with regard to childhood problems. There is an absence of large well-controlled, rigorously designed studies. Most evaluative work has been conducted on adults. Some theorists[23] claim that there are no differences between therapeutic approaches with regard to outcome. It is just such an assumption which leads some clinicians to argue that the effective factors are the same for all therapies and they can be identified with the common components of all types of influence and healing (warmth, respect, kindness, hope, understanding, provision of 'explanations').

Children are frequently referred to clinics for help with circumscribed problems such as enuresis, phobias, temper tantrums and the like. These are the types of problem which are most amenable to behaviour therapy.[39,40] There is some evidence[41] that an approach which educates significant adults in the child's environment is more effective than traditional psychotherapy. Behavioural techniques require a degree of control over the client's environment, something more easily achieved in the home and classroom with youngsters than with adults living in a more open-ended environment.

It is not possible to be dogmatic about the *exclusive* value of any one approach to childhood neuroses. Various methods appear to be effective with different problems (see reference 42 for a review). Studies by Rutter *et al.*[42] and Shepherd *et al.*[44] provide useful normative data for British children. The counselling of parents as to the normality of the children and indeed the 'normality' of many of their emotional problems, can produce a sense of relief and the calm and sensible handling which allows them to remain the transitory problems that they are when given sensible management.[5,30] What is also reassuring is the point made earlier in the chapter, that for the most part, neurotic children become reasonably well-adjusted adults; they are almost as likely to grow up 'normal' as children drawn at random from the general population.[44,45]

# References

1. Achenbach, T. M. and Edelbrock, C. S., 'The Classification of Child Psychopathology: A Review and Analysis of Empirical Efforts', *Psychological Bulletin*, **85** (1978), pp. 1275–301.
2. Macfarlane, J. W., Allen, L. and Honzik, M., *A Developmental Study of the Behaviour Problems of Normal Children* (University of California Press, Berkeley, 1954).
3. Erikson, E., *Childhood and Society* (revised edn) (Penguin Books, Harmondsworth, 1965).
4. Levitt, E. E., 'Research on Psychotherapy in Children', in A. E. Bergin and S. L. Garfield, (eds), *Handbook of Psychotherapy and Behaviour Change: An*

*Empirical Analysis* (Wiley, New York, 1971).

5. Herbert, M., *Emotional Problems of Development in Children* (Academic Press, London, 1974).

6. Horney, K., *Our Inner Conflicts* (Norton, New York, 1945).

7. Fenichel, O., *The Psychoanalytic Theory of Neurosis* (Routledge and Kegan Paul, London, 1945).

8. Wolpe, J. *Psychotherapy by Reciprocal Inhibition* (Stanford University Press, Stanford, Calif., 1958).

9. Jahoda, M., *Current Concepts of Positive Mental Health* (Basic Books, New York, 1958).

10. Lee, S. G. M. and Herbert, M. (eds), *Freud and Psychology* (Penguin Books, Harmondsworth, 1970).

11. Freud, S., *Analysis Terminable and Interminable. Collected Papers of Sigmund Freud*, vol. 5 (Basic Books, New York, 1959).

12. Freud, A., *The Psycho-analytic Treatment of Children* (Imago, London, 1946).

13. Axline, V., *Play Therapy: The Inner Dynamics of Childhood* (Houghton Mifflin, Boston, 1947).

14. Axline, V. M., *Dibs in Search of Self* (Gollancz, London, 1966).

15. Coopersmith, S., *The Antecedents of Self-Esteem* (W. H. Freeman, London, 1967).

16. Hewitt, L. E. and Jenkins, R. L., *Fundamental Patterns of Maladjustment: The Dynamics of their Origin* (Thomas, Springfield, Ill., 1946).

17. Jenkins, R. L., 'The Varieties of Children's Behavioural Problems and Family Dynamics', *American Journal of Psychiatry*, **124** (1968), pp. 1440–5.

18. Schaefer, E. S., 'A Circumplex Model for Material Behaviour', *Journal of Abnormal Social Psychology*, **59** (1959), pp. 226–35.

19. Becker, W. C., 'Consequences of Different Kinds of Parental Discipline', in M. L. Hoffman and L. W. Hoffman, (eds) *Review of Child Development Research*, vol. 1 (Russell Sage Foundation, New York, 1964), pp. 169–208.

20. Baumrind, D., 'Current Patterns of Parental Authority', *Developmental Psychology Monograph*, **4** (1) (1971), Pt. 2, pp. 1–103.

21. Herbert, M., *Conduct Disorders of Childhood and Adolescence: A Behavioural Approach to Assessment and Treatment* (John Wiley, Chichester, 1978).

22. Herbert, M. and Iwaniec, D., 'Behavioural Psychotherapy in Natural Home-settings: an Empirical Study Applied to Conduct Disordered and Incontinent Children', *Behavioural Psychotherapy*, **9** (1981), pp. 55–76.

23. Bergin, A. E. and Garfield, S. L. (eds), *Handbook of Psychotherapy and Behaviour Change* (John Wiley, Chichester, 1977).

24. Dollard, J. and Miller, N., *Personality and Psychotherapy* (McGraw-Hill, New York, 1950).

25. Alexander, F., 'The Dynamics of Psychotherapy in the Light of Learning Theory', *American Journal of Psychiatry*, **120** (1963), pp. 440–8.

26. Wachtel, P. L., *Psychoanalysis and Behaviour Therapy: Toward an Integration* (Basic Books, New York, 1977).

27. Murray, E. and Jacobson, L., 'The Nature of Learning in Traditional and Behavioural Psychotherapy', in A. Bergin and S. Garfield (eds) *Handbook of Psychotherapy and Behaviour Change: An Empirical Analysis* (Wiley, New York, 1971).

28. Erwin, E., *Behaviour Therapy: Scientific, Philosophical and Moral Foundations* (Cambridge University Press, Cambridge, 1978).

29. O'Leary, K. D. and Wilson, G. T., *Behaviour Therapy: Application and Outcome* (Prentice-Hall, Englewood Cliffs, New Jersey, 1975).

30. Herbert, M., *Behavioural Treatment of Problem Children: A Practice Manual* (Academic Press, London: Grune and Stratton, New York, 1981).

31. Kazdin, A. E., *History of Behaviour Modification: Experimental Foundations, of Contemporary Research* (University Park Press, Baltimore, 1978).

32. Bandura, A., *Principles of Behaviour Modification* (Holt, Rinehart and Winston, New York, 1969).

33. Bandura, A., *Social Learning Theory* (Prentice-Hall, Englewood Cliffs, New Jersey, 1977).

34. Rimm, D. C. and Masters, J. C., *Behaviour Therapy: Techniques and Empirical Findings* (Academic Press, New York, 1979).

35. Mathews, A., 'Fear-reduction Research and Clinical Phobias', *Psychological Bulletin*, **85** (2) (1978), pp. 390–404.

36. D'Zurilla, T. G. and Goldfried, M. R., 'Problem Solving and Behaviour Modification', *Journal of Abnormal Psychology*, **78** (1971), pp. 107–27.

37. Kendall, P. C., 'Cognitive-behavioural Interventions with Children' in B. Lahey and A. E. Kazdin (eds) *Advances in Child Clinical Psychology*, vol. 4 (Plenum Press, New York, 1981).

38. Meichenbaum, D., *Cognitive-Behaviour Modification: An Integrative Approach* (Plenum Press, London, 1977).

39. Gelfand, D. M. and Hartmann, D. P., *Child Behaviour: Analysis and Therapy* (Pergamon Press, Oxford, 1975).

40. Kazdin, A. E., 'Advances in Child Behaviour Therapy: Applications and Implications', *American Psychologist*, **34** (10) (1979), pp. 981–7 (Special Issue).

41. Donofrio, A. F., 'Parent Education and Child Psychotherapy', *Psychology in the Schools*, **13** (1976), pp. 176–80.

42. Rutter, M. and Hersov, L., *Child Psychiatry: Modern Approaches* (Blackwell, Oxford, 1977).

43. Rutter, M., Tizard, J. and Whitmore, K. (eds), *Education, Health and Behaviour* (Longmans Greens, London, 1970).

44. Shepherd, M., Oppenheim, B. and Mitchell, S., *Childhood Behaviour and Mental Health* (University of London Press, 1971).

45. Robins, L. N. and Lewis, R. G., 'The Role of the Antisocial Family in School Completion and Delinquency: A Three Generation Study', *Sociological Quarterly*, **1** (1966), pp.500–14.

# 12 PSYCHOTIC ANXIETY IN CHILDREN AND ITS TREATMENT

Timothy Telford Yates

## Introduction

It is not universally agreed upon as to what psychotic anxiety is or indeed, whether such a phenomenon exists.

In Hinsie and Campbell's *Psychiatric Dictionary* there is no entry under 'anxiety, psychotic'. However, their definition of 'panic' is more promising: '(panic is) . . . an attack of overwhelming anxiety . . . (which) . . . some writers restrict . . . to psychotic episodes, characterized by unrealistically based and autistically determined anxiety of overwhelming proportions.[1])

Even more directly relevant to this chapter, is the subsequent entry, 'panic, primordial':

> reactions of fright and anger combined with unfocused, disorganized, motor responses akin to the infantile startle reaction; such reactions are seen in many schizophrenic children. Primordial panic is also termed *elemental anxiety* and is believed to be based on primary self-awareness, and differentiation of the self from the nonself.[1]

Since the descriptions of 'panic' and of 'primordial panic' have been chosen as a working definition of psychotic anxiety it must be noted that such phrases as 'defects in the ego' and 'differentiation of self from non-self' are psychodynamic in origin. The reason that such phrases have been incorporated into the dictionary definition is perhaps because psychotic anxiety has been discussed most exhaustively by psychoanalysts and ego psychologists. Such a choice of language will necessarily influence the discussion.

To accept a psychodynamic frame of reference implies a *developmental* approach which carries with it certain basic assumptions.

Development presumes that the human organism is ever increasing in the complexity and organisation of its psychophysical structures and their functions. This implies that children become progressively more differentiated as they mature so that some phenomena which stand out as discrete entities in adulthood are not so well demarcated in children. Generally, the younger the child the more amorphous the phenomenon. Thus, anxiety, which may be sub-classified many ways in adults, becomes a more elusive concept in infants and pre-school children.

The use of the term 'anxiety' varies with the literature. Some authors speak of anxiety only as an *observable* phenomenon characterised by the obvious behavioural manifestations of extreme fear. Other authors use the term to describe something which may be *inferred* from such behaviours as withdrawal, sudden outbursts of rage, and so forth. These latter observers have often used the term with a developmental connotation which implies that a certain level of intrapsychic differentiation has been attained so as to allow for conflicts among the psychic structures (id, ego, and superego). These authors usually suggest that psychotic anxiety is not the same as neurotic or developmental anxiety since the former occurs before the ego is fully structured.

In passing, it is noteworthy that the words 'psychotic' and 'anxiety' are only infrequently juxtaposed in textbooks and journals and in scientific reference indices (such as Index Medicus). The words do not appear together on computer search programs such as MEDLINE and Psychological Abstracts. It may be that authors and compilers of data banks see little use in making a distinction between psychotic anxiety and any other type of anxiety. The issue as to whether psychotic anxiety is different in amount from other anxieties is one of the dominant themes of the literature.

## Essential Questions About Psychotic Anxiety

As we have seen, simply putting the words 'psychotic' and 'anxiety' together raises many questions.

What are the characteristics of (psychotic) anxiety? Is it fear of annihilation or of psychological disintegration as some have suggested? Further, what is experienced before one is aware that there is some *thing* to disintegrate or to be annihilated? What relationship do primitive anxieties have to psychotic anxiety? Does it differ qualitatively from neurotic or developmental anxiety or merely quantively? Can 'anxiety' only be experienced at a certain level of ego development? What is the role of object relationships in the genesis and treatment of psychotic anxiety? Is it experienced differently in children than it is in adults? Are there differences in anxiety among the different subtypes of childhood psychosis?

Finally, is anxiety central to the psychotic process or epiphenomenal?


## An Anxiety Hierarchy

A developmental orientation implies a hierarchy of anxieties which range from an ineffable, 'primordial' anxiety to more differentiated and more structured anxieties such as those associated with neurosis and developmental crises. A developmental sequence of anxiety is a necessary backdrop for a discussion of psychotic anxiety as a developmental phenomenon.

Among the earliest anxieties is fear of *loss of the 'object'* (significant person) to whom one is attached. More differentiated, and therefore presumably more developmentally advanced, is the fear of the loss of the love of this essential person. This latter kind of anxiety may arise for example during the so-called anal period wherein anxiety is generated around *loss of control of impulses* with the presumed consequence that the attachment to the all-powerful parent figure would be threatened. In psychodynamic terms *castration anxiety* is seen as being the pivotal event within the susequent Oedipal period for both boys and girls, although the anxiety is experienced differently in each sex. Psychoanalytical authors, such as Anna Freud, note that children of an oedipal age seem to have an upsurge of fears about bodily damage or injury. With the arrival of the oedipal situation and castration anxiety, the stage is set for neurotic anxiety about which little further will be said in this chapter, except to use it as a reference point of non-psychotic pathological anxiety with which its psychotic counterpart may be compared and contrasted.

But what is it that occurs *before* the fear of loss of the object?


## Characteristics of Psychotic Anxiety in Children

Thus, far, a definition has been proposed which implies a

developmental hierarchy of anxieties in which the earliest ones are profound and disorganised and the later ones conflict-based and structured. It is suggested that these developmentally primitive anxieties and psychotic anxiety are one and the same.

If psychotic anxiety is a discrete phenomenon it must be distinguishable from non-psychotic anxieties by observable and identifiable characteristics. Neurotic and developmental anxieties have been described and characterised by those who have suffered from them. Since psychotic children rarely can verbalise their terror, let us look at a primitive anxiety which appears closely to resemble psychotic anxiety but which seems more accessible ie anxiety in the Borderline child.

### Borderline Anxiety

This affect has been well described and shares characteristics both with primitive and with structured anxiety. Rosenfeld and Sprince wrote in 1963:

> the anxiety reactions we observed in . . . (borderline) . . . latency children and adolescents were intense, diffuse, panic-like, and seemed to involve the experience of disintegration and annihilation. It appeared as if the quality of the anxiety differed from that of the neurotic who experiences anxiety as a signal danger, the ego of the borderline child . . . cannot find appropriate measures to reduce the level of anxiety. Signal anxiety is therefore experienced as a threat which may lead to overwhelming feelings of disintegration.[2]

In psychodynamic terminology, signal anxiety functions as a warning to the ego that a threat is to be expected from within the organism in the form of an impending intrapsychic conflict. In response to this signal the ego mobilises defensive forces so as to minimise the impact of the assault. Rosenfeld and Sprince proposed that the defensive capacity of the borderline child's ego structure is not developmentally adequate to respond to the anxiety as a signal. Because the defences are so uncoordinated, primitive, and ill-structured, the child experiences a diffuse panic since the anxiety, intended as a signal, cannot be reduced in intensity by any of the normal defensive mechanisms nor 'bound' into a neurotic symptom.Rather, the signal anxiety *itself* becomes the threat.

It appears as if, in this type of child, anxiety is continually amplified in a sort of chain reaction. It is interesting, but perhaps moot, to speculate as to whether the signal anxiety triggers primordial anxiety or whether the experience of disintegration or annihilation is simply the result of a quantitatively overwhelming amount of anxiety made the greater because of the absence of defence.

> In some children, the anxiety seems to represent a reexperiencing of an infantile traumatic situation which took place when the ego was not sufficiently developed to deal with the overwhelming anxiety-provoking stimuli. This may . . . be connected with the observation . . . that some of our children have difficulty in inhibiting and selecting stimuli.[3]

These children seem to demonstrate a defect in maintaining the boundary between *self* and *other* both in a physical and in a psychological sense. This vagueness of psychological boundaries renders them easily prey to anxiety regarding loss of self and often related to an equally intense fear of actually *becoming* the other person. Either of these can give rise to feelings of annihilation. When annihilation anxieties are projected on to the environment they may be seen in borderline children as the catastrophic fear that the whole world is falling apart or being destroyed.

Because the boundaries between self and other are unclear in these children they cannot *internalise* the behaviour of others around them or even use those others to help screen and select relevant stimuli. Because of this defect in internalisation they are continually dependent upon the presence of an external object (another person). Equally hazy are the boundaries between thought and action. In borderline children, aggressive *thoughts* become easily equated with aggressive *acts* which can be particularly terrifying since such thoughts occur in the presence of severely impaired reality testing.

Rosenfeld and Sprince also suggest that there is a defect in the neutralisation of aggressive wishes which are often expressed directly since they are not neutralised nor defended against. In turn this arouses an intense fear of retaliation which may also be connected with anxiety about annihilation.[4]

## Psychotic Anxiety

Thomas Freeman suggests that psychotic children do not experience emotion as we understand it but rather are subject to a bombardment of peripheral (visceral, proprioceptive, tactile, etc.) sensations which he terms 'pre-emotional experiences'. He feels that this jumble of intense and disorganised affects can lead 'to an acute and intense anxiety which in turn results in serious acts of aggression'.[5] This view finds support from Ruth Thomas who feels that:

> confusions seem to arise in a futile attempt to organize organic and peripheral sensations to an abiding sense of the bodily self. They significantly lack the experience of emotional states with *specific quality* as we know them, and are characterized by an intense, diffuse form of excitement . . . accompanied by the most intense and ungovernable anxiety and give rise to aggressive reactions of great magnitude. Some children . . . are driven to . . . killing animals, some to violent attacks on themselves or others.[6]

In contradistinction to the idea of psychotic anxiety as a separate species of affect, others feel that the differences are not as profound. Fish and Ritvo feel that the issue is more quantitative than qualitative: 'Anxiety is a common symptom in many psychiatric disorders in children. Only the illogicality surrounding its eruption and its excessively unmodulated quality, distinguish the anxiety of psychotic children from that of less disturbed children.'[7]

Psychotic anxiety has a diffuse and chaotic quality which renders the sufferer utterly helpless. So too the timing and intensity of its eruption makes it appear utterly unpredictable from the point of view of an outside observer which makes it all the more frightening to *him* and may render him as helpless as the panicky child.

## Neurotic Anxiety

By contrast, children suffering from neurotic anxiety display clearer connections between people or situations and the onset of anxiety. In most instances the anxiety is modulated, bound, and usually comprehensible by an observer sensitive to the child's developmental tasks. Neurotic children are more prone to internalise: even when the conflict is externalised there is usually a discernable symbolic connection between the child, the symptom and often, the family system.

## Psychotic Anxiety and Ego Development

Although we have been making reference to issues of ego

development none is more fundamental than the distinction between *self* and *other*.

## Self-other Differentiation

The lack of this distinction is described particularly well by Margaret Mahler in what she came to call symbiotic psychosis.[8] The earliest ego is a 'body-ego'; the child's sense of its physical integrity and its physical boundaries. In some profoundly disturbed children it appears as if the boundaries of this body-ego are diffuse and so in turn are the boundaries of the psychological self. Many psychotic children seem to confuse self and other. For example, a psychotic child pretending or actually feeding a therapist may open and close its mouth as if *it* were the one being fed. At a more symbolic level this self/other confusion may be represented by reversal of pronouns.

## Whole-part Differentiation

Psychotic children tend to have difficulty dealing with people as if they were integral wholes. In ego-psychology terms, these relationships are 'part-object' relationships and are felt to be precursors to the 'object constancy' which is achieved in normal children by the age of three.[9] At this stage of the child's development, emotional investment in the internalised representation of a significant other person — the object — begins to become independent of the immediate gratification which that person offers. Prior to this, integrated (whole) entities are not internalised so that distinctions between part and whole are not clear. To a very disorganised child the loss of the *love* of the 'object' may be confused with the loss of the object itself.

Borderline children show similar phenomena but in a circumscribed fashion because of their more advanced ego development. Rosenfeld and Sprince describe a 13-year-old boy who was obsessed by the study of insects. When interrupted in prolonged ruminations about these insects he became subject to disorganising anxiety attacks. Unlike more psychotic children however, his reality testing remained intact in most other areas of his life.[10]

## Object Relations and Modulation of Drives

Because of the confusion between self and other, aggressive and libidinal impulses originating from within the child are often projected to outside. This projection may account both for avoidance of others and the occasional aggressive attack upon them so that object relationships can be perceived simultaneously as both dangerous and essential:

> Special qualities of the anxiety which appear in psychotic children showed that a danger situation is almost constantly present. The danger is entirely due to the heightened drive cathexis . . . lessened whenever an object relationship can be established . . . through which both drive satisfaction and drive control can be obtained. In turn this leads to the danger of object loss . . . (and) . . . a further danger is created by the fear of consequences of merging with the object.[11]

The psychotic/borderline child is caught between a rock and a hard place. Without the external 'other' as an auxiliary ego, the child's anxiety escalates beyond control because his failure to internalise whole objects has left an inadequate ego structure with which to modulate the anxiety. The child must fall back on incorporation, which is more primitive than internalisation, to form the necessary bond with the person acting as auxiliary ego. However, this represents a threat because it carries with it the fear of *merging* with the object and concomitant anxiety about annihilation. Incorporation of a part-object by a child whose boundaries between self and other are diffuse, may induce a terror of being 'swallowed up'. This is a common manifestation of annihilation anxiety.

### An Aetiological Hypothesis

Mahler feels that the pathology in the establishment of ego boundaries has its origins in a defective mother-child relationship.[12] She feels that the perceptual distortion so central to early-onset childhood psychosis arises out of a failure of ego structuralisation. Without such structuralisation, the child cannot become aware of itself as separate from others, i.e. 'individuate'. The failure of individuation in turn, occurs because the child is unable to master separation. If the distance between self and other is too great, the child fears it will fall apart. If the distance is not enough, the child fears it will be absorbed.

Either because of the child's constitutional limitations or the mother's inadequate parenting, no capacity for the child to acquire the ability to screen irrelevant from relevant stimuli was acquired. Psychotic children have an enormous difficulty separating 'signal' from 'noise' which renders them easily overwhelmed.

Under normal circumstances the mothering object is perceived as a *whole* object and then internalised, providing a nidus for further ego development.

> We believe that in cases of child psychosis the crucial disturbance has been the infant's lack or loss of the ability to utilize the mother during the early phases of life as a complement to, and organizer of, its own maturation. The result has been the absence of a human beacon of orientation, both in the world of reality and in his own inner world; from this has followed gross impairments of the integrating, synthesizing and organizing functions of the ego.[12]

In borderline children for example, these overwhelming stimuli may be dealt with by 'shifting levels of organisation' wherein regression produces a 'total shift to a more psychotic-like state', which successfully reduced the level of anxiety at the expense of the child's *total* adaptation to the environment. It is the absence of a finely tuned defensive structure which allows such global regression.[14]

### Anxiety in the Diagnosis of Childhood Psychosis

If anxiety is seen as being a pivotal event in childhood psychosis it is reasonable to expect that it will be clearly recognisable to an external observer. One would expect then, that anxiety would be an important criterion for the diagnosis of childhood psychosis in our nosological systems.

DSM III[15] holds that childhood psychoses bear little relationship to the adult psychoses. Child psychoses are grouped under the heading of Pervasive Developmental Disorders (excluding only schizophrenia, diagnosable by adult criteria).[15] In DSM III the Childhood Onset Pervasive Developmental Disorders list 'anxiety as one of seven signs/symptoms of which only three need be present for diagnosis'. According to this system anxiety is only variably observable in childhood psychoses.

The GAP diagnostic system[17] proposed that each childhood psychosis be grouped by its age of onset. These are than characterised as psychoses of: (1) infancy and early childhood (including

Symbiotic Psychosis); (2) later childhood; (3) adolescence.[16]

Kolvin *et al.* distinguishes three groups of childhood psychoses by age on onset: (1) onset before three years of age (Early-Onset); (2) onset from three to five years (Early-Onset); (3) onset after five (Later-Onset).[17]

Only in the first group did Kolvin[18] feel that the presence of anxiety was a significant discriminating variable. For the early onset groups he suggested using Kanner's[19] or Creak's criteria. Kanner commented on the anxiety generated by interference with an autistic child's environment[19] and the British Working Party,[20] which included Mildred Creak, wrote that 'frequent, acute, excessive, and seemingly illogical' anxiety is most commonly associated with separation or with environmental change.

Rutter *et al.*[21] in the proposed 'Classification Scheme for Psychiatric Disorders in Children and Adolescents', nowhere insists upon the presence of observable anxiety as being necessary for diagnosis of a psychosis.

By contrast, Goldfarb,[22,23] in discussing childhood schizophrenia (possibly analogous to Kolvin's Late-Onset group), spoke of a state of primordial anxiety found in this population. Loretta Bender[24] feels that anxiety is so characteristic of childhood schizophrenia that it is 'these children's first response and may be unremitting from the first day of life'. It is her feeling that increasingly manifest anxiety is a poor prognostic sign; one which heralds a personality disintegration. Writers on the subject of later-onset psychoses in children make reference rather to a 'blunting' or 'shallowness' of affect rather than an excess of anxiety.

In the *Basic Handbook of Child Psychiatry* is to be found a chart of 16 major authors on the subject of childhood psychosis of whom six felt that extreme anxiety was a significant contributor to the diagnosis of childhood psychoses; nine felt the symptom of anxiety was present, but not necessary for diagnosis; and one felt that anxiety or panic was 'rare' or 'not specific' to this disorder.[25]

It is difficult to make these various observations cohere. It may be that there is a lapse in the distinction made between the anxiety *observed* and anxiety *inferred*. For example, Janet Brown listed 'high anxiety' as present in 17 of 21 cases of children with Atypical Development yet ranked it twenty-third in a symptom list behind such behaviours as 'excluded stimuli', 'strong or unusual fears', 'diffuse aggression', and 'separation problems'.[26] Some dynamic theorists would infer the presence of anxiety in each of these higher ranking symptoms. The authors tend to see anxiety as being more prevalent in psychoses than phenomenologically based authors who demand *manifest* anxiety for diagnosis.

Anxiety is manifest in the autistic child when his obsession with 'sameness' is interfered with. In 'Symbiotic Psychosis' anxiety is most characteristic and specific for issues of separation. In the borderline, anxiety is described as frequent and dramatic; yet in DSM III (where these disorders have fallen under the heading of 'Schizotypal Personality Disorder') anxiety is not listed among the diagnostic criteria.

In summary, a child may be diagnosed as having a Pervasive Developmental Disorder or a Childhood Psychosis, at any age of onset before puberty, *without manifest* anxiety.

### Anxiety in Childhood and in Adult Psychoses

A developmental view of psychosis suggests that some of the phenomena of adult psychosis are regressive and may resemble some aspects of childhood psychosis, neurosis and even developmentally normal child behaviour.

This is particularly demonstrable in those adult psychoses with an acute onset and a short course which tend to be both disorganised and anxiety-filled. It is also true of chronic psychoses which are characterised by sudden, intense eruptions of affect. Thomas Freeman feels, in contradistinction to the authors of DSM III, that what the childhood and adult psychoses share most prominently is 'severe anxiety which frequently reaches a state of panic'.[27] Such psychotic adults seem to have the same self-perpetuating escalation of anxiety as has been described for borderline and psychotic children. Defences against such anxiety involve massive regression resulting in, for example, negativistic withdrawal or aggressive outbursts. 'In common with the children, adult patients dread the effect of their sexuality and aggression on others. They fear bodily disintegration and loss of personal, physical, and sexual identity.'[28]

There are also parallels in the psychological therapy of the psychoses of children and of adults. In each case the goal is to desensitise the patient to interpersonal contact by the measured formation of a relationship with a therapist. By virtue of this bond the therapist begins to help strengthen the patient's ego by becoming an auxiliary ego and thus allowing for internalisation. The structure thus offered helps the patient to deal with the next phase of therapy which involves relatively non-threatening interpretations of defensive manoeuvres which have hitherto obstructed the formation of mature relationships. The patient is helped to find alternative strategies which are more adaptive and developmentally appropriate.

## Particular Approaches to Psychotic Anxiety in Children

### Melanie Klein

Klein uses language and imagery delivered from adult psychoses to describe normal child development phenomena. She suggests that in infancy, children pass through a 'paranoid-schizoid position' and, in the latter half of the first year, a 'depressive postion'. During the first of these phases, the child's relationship is to part-objects, i.e. there is no internalised image of a whole, integrated person but rather a disconnected jumble of functions and features derived from the environment. There is a tendency to split 'good' from 'bad' which of course precludes an integrated perception of an other person who may be both good and bad at different times. The anxiety thus experienced is 'paranoid'. When the mother has begun to be recognised as a *whole*, the depressive position has begun and is characterised by greater integration but also by ambivalence, depressive anxiety and guilt.

In Melanie Klein's terminology 'position' implies:

a specific configuration of object relationships, anxieties and defenses which persist throughout life . . . Some paranoid and depressive anxieties always remain active within the personality but when the ego is sufficiently integrated and has established a relatively secure relationship to reality . . . neurotic mechanisms gradually take over from psychotic ones.[29]

It is difficult to summarise a theoretical position as complex as that of Melanie Klein. Nevertheless, most authors seem reluctant to use terminology derived from adult psychopathology to describe normal infantile emotional development. Her viewpoint suggests that psychosis emerging at any age, represents a developmental regression to positions which are universal and normative during the first year of life.

## Donald M. Winnicott

It is Winnicott's view that the personality in earliest infancy is unintegrated and that regressive disintegration leads back to this 'primary unintegration'.

> Ego mechanisms for defense . . . were assumed to be organized in relation to anxiety which derived either from instinct tension or object loss. This . . . presupposes a separateness of a self and a structuring of the ego . . . (which) . . . makes anxiety from instinct tension or object loss possible. Anxiety at this early stage . . . is, in fact, anxiety about annihilation.[30]

Winnicott speaks of a 'holding phase' of development which has the characteristics of primary process, primary identification, autoerotism, and primary narcissism. During this phase the ego changes from an unintegrated to an integrated state and the infant becomes able to experience anxiety about disintegration for the first time.[31] Prior to this change such anxiety was not able to be experienced because there was nothing that could *dis*integrate.

> Where annihilation, not castration anxiety is found as an important feature, then . . . (the) . . . diagnosis is not psychoneurosis, but psychosis. It is . . . a matter of whether the threat is in terms of a part object of a whole object . . . Just as a study of psychoneurosis leads a student to the oedipus complex . . . so the study of psychosis leads to the earliest stages of infant life.[32]

Presumably annihilation anxiety may arise during the holding phase when the ego changes from an unintegrated to an integrated state. Whether one can speak of 'anxiety' *before* that has happened is debatable. It is nevertheless clear that Winnicott sees a direct connection between adult psychosis and infantile development processes.

## The Treatment of Psychotic Anxiety

### General Principles

Ruttenberg and Angert outlined five principles of treatment dealing with psychotic children.[33]

Because of 'a growing trend towards a concept of multicausality' they believe that therapy of psychotic children requires a multi-disciplinary approach. The protean nature of childhood psychosis precludes a single treatment approach and no individual is capable of meeting the complete range of the psychotic child's needs.

Secondly, the child must be approached at its developmental level, regardless of chronological age or physical size.

Next, programmes for such children must reach beyond the intrinsic behaviour into the child's larger environment and his living situation. Involvement of parents and families in treatment is strongly emphasised.

So too, the treatment plan must be continually revised in order to keep pace with the evolution of the child's disorder or its changing nature in response to treatment. 'The child who progresses from a state of autistic withdrawal to a symbiotic stage of clinging attachment to a more schizophrenic-type of illness, will need somewhat different therapeutic approaches at each stage and emphasis may be switched from one therapist to another'.

Finally, no less than a three year trial of treatment should be attempted before the resources are withdrawn and the assumption made that further progress is unlikely.

There are some, most prominently Bruno Bettleheim, who feel that such children are best separated from their parents in order to facilitate treatment.[34,35] More recently, Schopler and Reichler have demonstrated that early and continued involvement of the parents as co-therapists is productive and useful.[36]

Although many theorists suggest that anxiety around earliest interpersonal relationships produced an initial failure of internalisation, it has not been suggested that elimination of psychotic anxiety will, of *itself*, produce a reversal of the pathology. In early-onset psychoses, if there is no manifest anxiety in the child's behaviour, there is little evidence that the use of specific anti-anxiety treatment will play other than an adjunctive role in the treatment plan.

One the other hand, in the treatment of late-onset psychoses and those earlier onset psychoses where manifest anxiety *is* present, its alleviation is often considered essential to further progress, which usually involves other modalities of therapy. A variety of methods have been offered to deal with such anxiety as it arises.

*Medication*

In the early-onset psychoses, anxiolytic medication is indicated for manifest anxiety interfering with ongoing treatment.

In most cases of childhood psychosis, phenothiazines have been found helpful in controlling episodes of panic or 'disintegrative' anxiety.[37] Relief of such anxiety enhances the psychotherapeutic reconstruction of the ego since it supports existing defensive functions and allows the child a greater capacity to tolerate intimacy with others.

Of this family of drugs, chlorpromazine and thioridazine have been found to be most helpful in controlling panic, in part because of their sedative properties.[38,39] Haloperidol has also been found useful in controlling acute psychotic episodes where, presumably, the prevalence of high-anxiety symptomatology is greater than in those cases where the onset is more insidious.[40]

Apart from major tranquillisers, the only other medication recommended to control anxiety and restlessness in psychotic children is diphenylhydramine.[41]

Minor tranquillisers of the benzodiazepine family have usually been reported to be ineffective or actively harmful in the treatment of psychotic children.[42] It is difficult to draw any far-reaching conclusions about the role of anxiety in childhood psychoses from the variable effectiveness of these specifically anxiolytic medications. One notes that minor tranquillisers have been found to be of only equivocal use even in the anxiety of neurotic children.

An interesting variation however, is the opinion offered by Klein in talking about adult psychoses.

> Ineffectiveness of chlorpromazine in the anxious patient indicated that this drug should not be conceptualized as an antianxiety drug but because chlorpromazine was effective in the schizophrenic (who must be exceedingly anxious) and ineffective or toxic in the anxious patient meant that the anxiety of these patients was not simply less than that of psychotic patients. Therefore the continuity theory, which held that psychosis was simply a quantitative spilling over of the same anxiety suffered by people in more moderate disorders, could not be correct. If anything, the situation implied a physiological discontinuity.[43]

## Psychotherapy and Family Therapy

The building of relationships with psychotic children, usually in the context of a structured milieu, has long been seen as the cornerstone of ego-restorative efforts. Anxiety-reducing techniques in therapy include the therapist's continual adjustment to the regressed state of the child since for example, the child's primitive defensive structure, in its vulnerability, may interpret as a threat what might seem like a well-meaning advance or a desirable treat to a normal adult.

All efforts toward lifting a child from his psychosis are devoted to establishing an enduring emotional bond with another human being. 'There is only room for one person in a psychosis. As soon as two people are in, there is a cure, providing . . . that one of them realizes the difference between inner and outer realities.'[44] Insofar as anxiety impedes the formation of this attachment, it must be dealt with as a matter of priority.

Therapists from a psychoanalytic background are often more active in making verbal interpretations of the child's inner state. Analysts see the essential goal as the restoration of ego functions, object relation and the neutralisation of aggressive forces by libidinal gratification. Along with interpretation, emphasis is placed on the function of the therapist as auxiliary ego and setter of limits. The auxiliary ego function is seen as restoring the availability of the first maternal person as giver of structure and allowing for a renewed opportunity to internalise a 'filter' of external stimuli.

No matter what sort of psychotherapy is brought to bear, it is clear that the remainder of the child's environment must be highly structured.

## Milieu Therapy

Virtually all treatment programmes for psychotic children demand an environment which *actively* provides structure for the child. This controls the anxiety by limiting the stimuli and by setting appropriate limits as well as by bringing to bear a variety of techniques to break the cycle of anxiety once begun. The milieu learns to buffer the child against threatening stimuli which requires intimate knowledge of the child's idiosyncratic responses to particular stimuli. Well-trained adults learn to maintain an optimal distance between themselves and such children and to reduce these distances in a measured way. In this way the child may become accustomed to an 'other' so as to minimise fears of merger or attack.

Since there are many accounts of milieux designed to treat

psychotic children there is no need to describe them here. With respect to the treatment of psychotic anxiety in particular, the thrust of any milieu must be to maintain a balance between over-stimulating the child so as to produce counter-therapeutic anxiety and being so undemanding as to avoid *any* anxiety and thus pose no challenge for ego growth.

## Behaviour Modification

Behavioural techniques are invariably integral to a structured milieu for psychotic children but they have other more specific applications as well.

Graziano and Kean have successfully taught psychotic children techniques of muscular relaxation in spite of earlier opinions that this was not possible. They originally found that reciprocal inhibition was virtually ineffective with psychotic children since the anxiety was much less focused than in other diagnostic categories. They discovered then that there was not only a decrease of the excitement response during the relaxation training itself but also that this calming effect persisted throughout the whole day. The planned second phase of therapy, systematic desensitisation, was often unnecessary because of the relatively spectacular effect of the relaxation training.[45]

## Concluding Remarks

Psychotic anxiety is distinguishable from its neurotic counterpart by its suddenness of onset, its exaggerated intensity, its self-perpetuating escalation, its ego-disruptive qualities, and its profound capacity to produce global regression. Because of these characteristics it is highly resistant to either medical or to psycho-therapeutic attempts to ameliorate it.

Psychotic anxiety can be understood developmentally but it is qualitatively different for neurotic or developmental anxiety. With the beginning formation of a more complete ego structure in the second half of the first year of life, the defensive structure allows for the experience of anxiety around merger of annihilation. Before that, it is questionable whether affects are sufficiently dif-ferentiated to speak of the term 'anxiety' at all.

The quality of anxiety in adult psychoses, particularly those of acute onset or characterised by severe exacerbations, seems similar to that found in the childhood psychoses. Continuity with developmental or neurotic anxiety is more questionable.

The defect from which childhood psychoses originate seems to arise from the early relationship between the infant and the maternal person. In some instances this deficiency may arise from a deeply flawed environment whereas in others a 'good enough' environment has been provided but seems to have had little impact on a child because constitutional limitations have not permitted the child to respond to normal ministrations. If we accept the view that childhood psychoses are multicausal then there are those children whose disorders spring primarily from a disturbance of nature and others from a disturbance of nurture. Since we are interactional beings from birth however, it is still difficult to disentangle biological predispositions from learned behaviours.

In response to the question as to whether anxiety is central to childhood psychosis or epiphenomenonal, an adequate reply has not been found. By the requirements of most nosological systems, it can be said that observable, manifest anxiety is *not* essential for the diagnosis of childhood psychosis. This may be merely a semantic issue wherein anxiety goes by another name so that, for example, aggressive manifestations might be recognised as manifestations of anxiety by one researcher and seen as utterly unrelated to anxiety by another.

*It is essential however, to regard manifest anxiety as a gauge to monitor the child's response to the environment and to provide clues as to points of vulnerability. So too, it is an important governor of the speed with which change is introduced and ego growth promoted.* Anxiety tells us when we are touching the child's inner core and regardless of the role that it plays in the *genesis* of childhood psychoses it is certain to be encountered as the child begins to emerge from his psychotic cocoon.

Anxiety must be continually managed so as to allow the child's defective ego structure to strengthen itself at an optimal pace. This demands that the therapist continually help to maintain sufficient structure within the child so as to prevent his being overwhelmed by anxiety. At the same time the therapist must avoid smothering necessary anxiety arising from a developmental challenge which must be met for growth to take place.

It is in maintaining this balance that the art of treating psychotic children reaches its fullest expression.

## References

1. Hinsie, L. E. and Campbell, R. J. (eds), *Psychiatric Dictionary* (4th ed) (Oxford University Press, New York, 1970), p. 526.

2. Rosenfeld, S. and Sprince, M., 'An Attempt to Formulate the Meaning of the Concept of "Borderline" ', *Psychoanalytic Study of the Child*, vol. 20 (1963), pp. 628−9.

3. Ibid., p. 629.

4. Ibid., pp. 615−29.

5. Freeman, T., *A Psychoanalytic Study of the Psychoses* (International Universities Press, New York, 1973), p. 312.

6. Thomas, R., 'Comments on Some Aspects of Self and Object Representation in a Group of Psychotic Children', *The Psychoanalytic Study of the Child*, vol. 21 (International Universities Press, New York, 1966), p. 549.

7. Fish, B. and Ritvo, E. R., 'Psychoses of Childhood' in J. D. Noshpitz (ed.), *Basic Handbook of Child Psychiatry*, vol. 2 *Disturbances in Development* (Basic Books, New York, 1979), p. 215.

8. Mahler, M. S. and Gosliner, B. J., 'On Symbiotic Childhood Psychosis', *The Psychoanalytic Study of the Child*, vol. 10 (International Universities Press, New York, 1955), pp. 195−212.

9. Mahler, M., 'On the Significance of the Normal Separation-Individuation Phase with Reference to Research in Symbiotic Childhood Psychosis' in M. Schur (ed.), *Drives, Affects, Behaviour* (International Universities Press, New York, 1965), pp. 161−99.

10. Rosenfeld, S. and Sprince, M., 'An Attempt to Formulate the Meaning of the Concept of "Borderline" ', *Psychoanalytic Study of the Child*, vol. 20 (1963), pp. 612−13.

11. Freeman, T., *A Psychoanalytic Study of the Psychoses* (International Universities Press, New York, 1973), p. 312.

12. Mahler, M. S. and Furer, M., 'Child Psychosis: A Theoretical Statement and its Implications', *Journal of Autism and Childhood Schizophrenia*, 2(3) (1972), pp. 213−81.

13. Ibid., p. 214.

14. Pine, F., 'On the Concept of "Borderline" in Children' in *Psychoanalytic Study of the Child* (International Universities Press, New York, 1974), pp. 350−2.

15. American Psychiatric Association, *Diagnostic and Statistical Manual of Mental Disorders* (DSM III) (Washington, D.C., 1980), pp. 35−99.

16. Group for the Advancement of Psychiatry, 'Psychopathological Disorders in Childhood: Theoretical Considerations and a Proposed Classification System', vol. VI, Report no. 62, June 1966, pp. 251−8.

17. Kolvin, I., 'Studies in the CHildhood Psychoses, I Diagnostic Criteria and Classification', *British Journal of Psychiatry*, 118 (1971), pp. 381−4.

18. Kolvin, I., Ounsted, C., Humphrey, M. and McNay, A., 'Studies in the Childhood Psychoses, II The Phenomenology of Childhood Psychoses', *British Journal of Psychiatry*, 118 (1971), pp. 385−95.

19. Kanner, L., 'Autistic Disturbance of Affective Contact', *Nervous Child*, 2 (1943), pp. 217−50.

20. Creak, M. *et al.*, 'Schizophrenic Syndrome in Children: Progress Report of the British Working Party', *British Medical Journal*, 2 (1961), pp. 889−90.

21. Rutter, M., Lebovici, S., Eisenberg, L. *et al.*, 'World Health Organization: A Triaxial Classification of Mental Disorders in Childhood', *Journal of Child Psychology and Psychiatry*, 10 (1969), pp. 41−61.

22. Goldfarb, W., *Childhood Schizophrenia* (Harvard University Press, Cambridge, Mass, 1961).

23. Goldfarb, W., 'Self-Awareness in Schizophrenic Children', *Archives of General Psychiatry*, **8** (1963), pp. 47–60.

24. Bender, L., 'Childhood Schizophrenia', *The Psychiatric Quarterly*, **4** (1953), p. 675.

25. Fish, B. and Ritvo, E. R., 'Psychoses of Childhood' in J. D. Noshpitz (ed.) *Basic Handbook of Child Psychiatry*, vol. II *Disturbances in Development* (Basic Books, New York, 1965), pp. 270–1.

26. Brown, J. L., 'Prognosis from Presenting Symptoms of Pre-school Children With Atypical Development', *American Journal of Orthopsychiatry*, XXX (2) (April 1960), p. 386.

27. Freeman, T., 'Childhood Psychopathology and Psychotic Phenomena in Adults', *British Journal of Psychiatry*, **124** (1974), pp. 560.

28. Freeman, T., *A Psychoanalytic Study of the Psychoses* (International Press, New York, 1973), p. 313.

29. Segal, H., *Introduction to the Work of Melanie Klein* (Hogarth Press and the Institute of Psychoanalysis, London, 1978), pp. vii–ix.

30. Winnicott, D. M., 'Parent-Infant Relationships (1960)', paper reprinted in 'The Maturational Processes and the Facilitating Environment' in J. D. Sutherland (ed.) *The International Psycho-analytic Library* (Hogarth Press, 1972), p. 41.

31. Ibid., p. 44.

32. Ibid., p. 130.

33. Ruttenberg, B. A. and Angert, A. J., 'Psychotic Disorders' in G. P. Sholevar *et al.* (eds), *Emotional Disorders in Children and Adolescents* (Spectrum Publications, Jamaica, New York, 1980), pp. 421–2.

34. Bettleheim, B., *The Empty Fortress: Infantile Autism and the Birth of the Self* (Free Press, New York, 1967).

35. Bettleheim, B., *A Home for the Heart* (Knopf, New York, 1974).

36. Schopler, E. and Reichler, R. J., 'Parents as Co-therapists in the Treatment of Psychotic Children', *Journal of Autism and Childhood Schizophrenia*, **1** (1970), pp. 87–102.

37. Ruttenberg, B. A. and Angert, A. J., 'Psychotic Disorders' in G. P. Sholevar *et al.* (eds), *Emotional Disorders in Children and Adolescents* (Spectrum Publications, Jamaica, New York, 1980), p. 445.

38. White, J. H., *Paediatric Psychopharmacology* (Williams and Wilkins Company, Baltimore, 1977), pp. 134–40.

39. Weiss, G., 'Child Psychopharmacology' in D. V. S. Sankar (ed.) *Psychopharmacology of Childhood* (PJD Publications, Westbury, New York, 1976), pp. 134–5.

40. White, J. H., *Paediatric Pharmacology* (Williams and Wilkins Company, Baltimore, 1977), p. 43.

41. Campbell, M., 'Biological Interventions in Psychoses of Childhood', *Journal of Autism and Childhood Schizophrenia*, **3** (4) (1973), p. 354.

42. Ibid.

43. Klein, D. F., 'Anxiety Reconceptualized' in D. F. Klein and J. G. Rabkin (eds) *Anxiety: New Research and Changing Concepts*, American Psychopathological Series (Raven Press, New York, 1981), p. 235.

44. Sandford, J. A., *Healing and Wholeness* (Paulist Press, New York, 1977), p. 83.

45. Graziano, A. M. and Kean, J. E., 'Programmed Relaxation and Reciprocal Inhibition with Psychotic Children', *Behavioural Research and Therapy*, **6** (1968), pp. 433–7.

There are a number of other articles pertaining to anxiety in psychotic children which were not included in the text of this chapter but are offered as a supplement to those who wish to delve further into the topic.

## General Works

1. Werry, J. S. and Aman, M. G., 'Anxiety in Children' in G. D. Burrows and B. Davies (eds) *Handbook of Studies of Anxiety* (Elsevier/North-Holland Biomedical Press, Amsterdam, 1980), pp. 165–92.

## Specific Papers

1. Misès, R. and Horrassius, M., 'Les Dysharmonies Evolutives Precoces de Structure Psychotique', *Revue de Neuropsychiatrie Infantile*, **21**(12) (1973), pp. 755–65.

2. Remschmidt, H., 'Observations on the Role of Anxiety in Neurotic and Psychotic Disorders at an Early Age', *Journal of Autism and Childhood Schizophrenia*, **3**(2) (1973), 00 106–14.

3. Campbell, M. *et al.*, 'The Effects of Haloperidol on Learning and Behaviour on Autistic Children', *Journal of Autism and Developmental Disorders*, **12**(2) (1982), p. 167.

Volume III of the *Basic Handbook of Child Psychiatry*, of which volume II is referred to in the text, contains helpful chapters on therapy of anxiety in childhood psychosis.

# INDEX